#18236487.

ML

7/ MAy

Spine

Spinal Imaging: Diagnostic and Therapeutic Applications

John H. Bisese, M.D.
Guest Editor

2 9 JAN 1997

STATE OF THE ART REVIEWS

Volume 2/ Number 3 May 1988
HANLEY & BELFUS, INC.-Philadelphia

Publisher: HANLEY & BELFUS, INC.
210 South 13th Street
Philadelphia, PA 19107

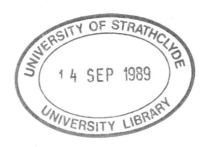

SPINE: State of the Art Reviews
May 1988 Volume 2, Number 3

ISSN 0887-9869
ISBN 0-932883-57-5

SPINE: State of the Art Reviews is published triannually (three times per year) by Hanley &
Belfus, Inc., 210 South 13th Street, Philadelphia, Pennsylvania 19107.

POSTMASTER: Send address changes to SPINE: State of the Art Reviews, Hanley & Belfus,
Inc., 210 South 13th Street, Philadelphia, PA 19107

This issue is Volume 2, Number 3.

The Editor of this publication is Linda C. Belfus.

The subscription price is $75.00 per year U.S., $87.00 per year outside U.S. (add $24.00 for
air mail). Single issues $32.00 U.S., $36.00 outside U.S. (add $8.00 for single issue air mail).

Evaluation of Posterior Spinal Structures by Computed Tomography
Ay-Ming Wang, David P. Wesolowski, and Jalil Farah

High-resolution CT allows excellent noninvasive evaluation of the bone and adjacent soft tissues of the spine. CT assessment of disorders of posterior spinal structures, including degenerative changes, spinal stenosis, trauma, primary bone neoplasm, metastatic disease, inflammatory process, spondylolysis, spondylolisthesis, and congenital anomalies are reviewed and illustrated.

Spinal Dysraphism: Evaluation by Myelography and Computed Tomography
Rebecca I. Ayres

Spinal dysraphism comprises disorders ranging in severity from spina bifida with widening of the dural sac to complex malformations such as myelomeningocele with hydromyelia and the Chiari malformation. In institutions in which MRI is not available, and for patients for whom MRI is inconclusive or technically inadequate, myelography and CT continue to play a major role in evaluating the patient with spinal dysraphism.

Evaluation of Spinal Dysraphism by Magnetic Resonance Imaging
John H. Bisese

The role of MRI in the evaluation of 50 patients with spinal dysraphism is discussed and illustrated. MRI offers an excellent alternative to CT and myelography, and takes considerably less time. The advantages of MRI over ionizing forms of imaging are discussed, especially the applicability of its multiplanar capacity in spinal dysraphic syndromes.

Magnetic Resonance Imaging of the Spine and Spinal Cord Tumors
Alan R. Alexander

Magnetic resonance imaging has many clear advantages over other available modalities in the evaluation of the spine and spinal cord for tumors and tumor-like conditions, and is currently considered by many authorities to be the modality of choice. The use of MRI in the diagnosis of intramedullary, extramedullary intradural, and extramedullary extradural tumors is discussed.

Evaluation of Disc Disease by Magnetic Resonance Imaging
William W. Woodruff

The application of MRI represents an evolutionary advance in the ability to evaluate patients with disc disease. Using slight differences in the proton density, and T1 and T2 relaxation times of various tissues, MRI allows multiplanar visualization of discs, cerebrospinal fluid, cord, and the perimeter of the spinal canal without the use of intravenous contrast material.

CONTENTS

CONTRIBUTORS

Alan R. Alexander, M.D.
Division of Neuroradiology, Department of Radiology, St. Joseph Hospital and Health Care Center, Lancaster, Pennsylvania

Rebecca I. Ayres, M.D.
Department of Radiology, Scottish Rite Children's Hospital, Atlanta, Georgia

M.O. Barth, M.D.
Service de Neuroradiology, Hopital Henri Mondor, Creteil, France

John H. Bisese, II, M.D.
Georgia Baptist Medical Center and Atlanta Magnetic Imaging, Atlanta, Georgia

Jalil Farah, M.D.
Clinical Associate Professor of Radiology, University of Michigan Medical School; Director of Diagnostic Radiology, William Beaumont Hospital, Royal Oak, Michigan

Richard W. Foster, M.D.
Assistant Professor of Radiology, Tulane University Medical Center, New Orleans, Louisiana

A. Gaston, M.D.
Service de Neuroradiology, Hopital Henri Mondor, Creteil, France

Barry F. Jeffries, M.D.
Georgia Baptist Medical Center, Atlanta, Georgia

F. Le Bras, M.D.
Service de Neuroradiology, Hopital Henri Mondor, Creteil, France

Theresa C. Power, D.O.
Neuroradiologist, Thomas Jefferson University Hospital, Philadelphia, Pennsylvania, and Mercy Catholic Medical Center, Darby, Pennsylvania

Barry M. Tom, M.D.
Resident, Radiology, Mercy Catholic Medical Center, Darby, Pennsylvania

James K. Wallman, M.D.
Neuroradiologist, Department of Radiology, Lahey Clinic Medical Center, Burlington, Massachusetts

Ay-Ming Wang, M.D.
Assistant Professor of Radiology, Harvard Medical School, and Brigham and Women's Hospital, Boston, Massachusetts

David P. Wesolowski, M.D.
Chief, Division of Neuroradiology, William Beaumont Hospital, Royal Oak, Michigan

William W. Woodruff, Jr., M.D., Major, USAF, MC
Department of Radiology, Wilford Hall USAF Medical Center, Lackland Air Force Base, Texas

PUBLISHED ISSUES 1986–1988

FUTURE ISSUES 1988–1989

Subscriptions and single issues available from the publisher—Hanley & Belfus, Inc., Medical Publishers, 210 South 13th Street, Philadelphia PA 19107 (215) 546-7293.

PREFACE

Roentgenographic and other imaging techniques are a potent ally in the diagnosis and management of spinal diseases and disorders. Modern imaging examinations frequently are an essential element in the formation of a diagnosis and often provide assistance during therapeutic procedures as well as information about the response to therapy.

Although some imaging modalities, such as ultrasound, have limited use and others are being replaced or changing position in the sequence of examinations, practically the full gamut of imaging technologies has some applicability to diagnosis and management of the multitude of problems that beset the spine, either as primary diseases and disorders or as a result of other systemic afflictions. Plain film examination is still often the initial step, but the roles of computed tomography and magnetic resonance are growing exponentially and in many instances they are already the leading modalities in the work-up of spinal disease. Other important procedures and imaging techniques include tomography, angiography, nuclear medicine scans, myelography, and thermography.

In this issue of **SPINE: State of the Art Reviews,** we have heavily emphasized the roles of CT and MRI, which continue to reshape the approach to spinal imaging and are subject to intensive research and study as new applications unfold. Also included are techniques that are partially therapeutic, such as epidural and facet injections, but that also yield a significant amount of diagnostic information and, in terms of invasiveness, are relatively low risk in the hands of an experienced clinician.

We also have the pleasure of including a contribution on "Spinal Angiography" from Dr. Wallman, who has acquired an unusual amount of interventional experience with Dr. Le Bras and associates from Creteil, France.

We believe we have assembled a useful issue of this series that should provide a good review for those already sophisticated in the various imaging modalities that apply to the spine and a helpful introduction for those who intend to become familiar with the state of the art of the diagnosis and treatment of spinal diseases and disorders.

JOHN BISESE, MD
GUEST EDITOR

vii

F. LE BRAS, MD[1]
J. WALLMAN, MD[2]
M.O. BARTH, MD[1]
A. GASTON, MD[1]

SPINAL ANGIOGRAPHY

[1]Service de Neuroradiology, Hopital Henri Mondor, Creteil, France

[2]Department of Diagnostic Radiology, Lahey Clinic Medical Center, Burlington, Massachusetts

Reprint Requests to:
James K. Wallman, M.D.
Lahey Clinic Medical Center
Department of Diagnostic
Radiology
41 Mall Road
Burlington, MA 01805

Since the initial description of spinal angiography more than 20 years ago by Djindjian in France and Di Chiro in the United States, there has been progress on many fronts: improvement in the understanding of the anatomical substrate; considerable improvement in the radiologic apparatus; development of new catheters; and development of new contrast materials that are much less toxic.

This article discusses the vascular anatomy of the spine and spinal cord, the angiographic technique, and the indications for treatment by the endovascular route.

ANATOMICAL CONSIDERATIONS

We will commence our discussion of the arterial supply to the spinal cord by describing the blood supply to the dorsal aspect of the spine in general. Because the cervical region is somewhat anomalous we will start with a general appreciation of the vascular anatomy of the dorsal and lumbar spines.

The thoracic and lumbar spine blood supply is fed by branches from the intercostal and lumbar arteries. (Figs. 1 and 2).[2,3] Branches of the trunk of the intercostal artery supply the anterior and lateral faces of the vertebral body. The branches originate before the bifurcation into the anterior intercostal artery and dorsal spinal artery. Commonly there are anastomotic branches oriented vertically between adjacent intercostal arteries. The anterior intercostal artery supplies the costotransverse articulation or the transverse apophyseal region. The dorsal spine artery supplies the interior surface of the

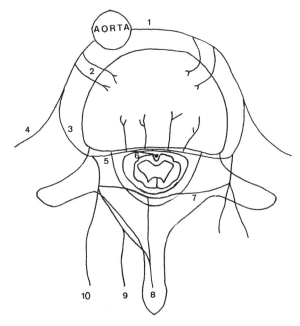

FIGURE 1. Vascular territory of the aortic intercostals. Bird's eye view of aorta, vertebral body, and blood vessels. 1. intercostal artery; 2. anterior vertebral body artery; 3. posterior or dorsospinal branch; 4. anterior intercostal artery; 5. posterior vertebral body or radiculo-medullary artery; 6. anterior radiculo-medullary artery; 7. prelaminar artery; 8, 9, 10. muscular branches.

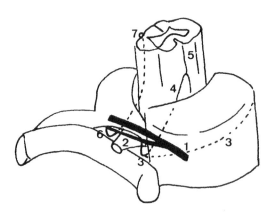

FIGURE 2. Origin and course of the radiculo-medullary arteries. Anterior lateral view of vertebral body, spinal cord, and vessels (dotted lines are arteries hidden by overlying structures). 1. intercostal artery; 2. posterior branch; 3. radiculo-medullary branch; 4. anterior radiculo-medullary artery; 5. anterior spinal artery; 6. posterolateral radiculo-medullary artery; and 7. posterior spinal artery.

spinal canal and contents. Supply to the posterior aspect of the vertebral body is via the anterior spinal canal branch, which forms collaterals over the posterior surface of the vertebral body in an "H" pattern. Further branching produces the anterior radiculo-medullary artery, destined to supply the spinal cord and meninges, while a posterior spinal canal branch supplies the dural surface of the lamina. Finally, the dorsal spine artery has spinal branches that supply the posterior aspect of the dura,[3] some of the posterior elements, and the paraspinal muscles and tendons.

The anterior four fifths of the spinal cord[7] is supplied by the anterior spinal artery, which lies in the anterior median fissure. Posteriorly, the posterior spinal arteries are paired structures situated in the lateral fissures, just posterior to the dorsal nerve roots. These supply only a part of the posterior columns and horns. In the cervical region the anterior spinal artery consists of branches ascending and descending from anterior radiculo-medullary spinal arteries originating from the subclavian arteries. There are many variations of this supply. In the dorsal and dorsal-lumbar region the anterior spinal artery originates from the inter-costals and lumbar arteries as mentioned above. In fact, the anterior radiculo-medullary spinal arteries are relatively few in number. It appears that in the course of development in the embryo the majority of the 62 radicular arteries regress. Thus the anastomotic possibilities are very limited. The two posterior spinal arteries, on the other hand, are of much less functional significance; however, there are many anastomotic branches from the posterior radiculo-medullary spinal arteries.

Anterior Spinal Artery

The anterior spinal artery begins in the region of C2 by the union of two descending branches from the terminal portion of the vertebral arteries. At the level of C3 or C4 it is joined by one or two anterior radiculo-medullary spinal arteries from the midcervical vertebral arteries and further down by a large radiculo-medullary artery, the artery of the cervical enlargement of Lazorthes, most commonly having its origin in the deep cervical branch of the thyrocervical trunk. Finally there are many arterial variations as to number, side, and origin at the C5, C6, and C7 levels, being usually from the costocervical trunk or first intercostals. The anterior spinal artery is not of uniform caliber throughout, being larger near the radiculo-medullary branches and smaller above and between them. This leads to relative "watershed" areas of diminished blood supply.

In the thoracic region the third or fourth intercostal artery, usually on the left, furnishes a radiculo-medullary branch to the anterior spinal artery, which never anastomoses with the descending branch of the artery of the cervical enlargement.[8]

The thoracolumbar spinal cord receives its major supply from the largest radiculomedullary branch, usually originating on the left side (75%), between D8 and D12 (likewise, 75% of the time). This is the so-called artery of Adamkiewicz. In the conus region there exist two anterior spinal branches that anastomose with the posterior spinal branches and are called the "arterial loop of the lumbar enlargement of Lazorthes." This important network is also sup-plied by the sacral radicular arteries, either the iliolumbar artery of the hypo-gastric artery or directly from the distal aorta.

The posterior spinal arteries begin in the cervical region from descending branches of the posterior inferior cerebellar arteries and surprisingly receive radiculo-medullary supply at nearly every intercostal level. Infrequently there is anastomosis of the anterior and posterior spinal arteries via circumferential branches.

Collaterals

In the high cervical region, in cases of obstruction of the vertebral or subclavian arteries, the collateral supply to the anterior spinal artery is via an anastomotic group called the "retroatlanto axial artery of Bosniak," formed by the muscular branches of the vertebral arteries, deep cervical arteries, ascending cervical arteries, the occipital branch of the external carotid arteries, and, finally, the posterior inferior cerebellar arteries.

In the low cervical region collateral supply is from the superior and inferior thyroidal arteries, the internal mammary arteries as well as the muscular branches of the vertebral arteries, deep cervical arteries, and ascending cervical arteries. There are no constant collaterals for the high thoracic spinal cord. The dorsolumbar spinal cord, however, has many possible collaterals via lumbosacral radicular arteries, which supply branches to the cone-shaped network (Lazorthes) formed by the union of the posterior spinal arteries with the artery of Adamkiewicz (see Fig. 5).

The Intramedullary Distribution

The interior of the spinal cord is divided into two large regions (central and peripheral) according to blood supply. The central arterial group has its supply from the anterior spinal artery, which is situated in the anterior median fissure, giving branches to the paramedian spinal tracks directly, and in the depths of the sulcus giving sulco-commissural branches to the gray substance. This network irrigates the anterior two thirds to four fifths of the spinal cord. The peripheral cord is supplied by penetrating branches from the circumferential (vasa corona) network formed by anastomotic branches of the three vertically oriented spinal arteries and the anterior and two posterior spinal arteries, forming so-called internal spinal arteries.

Venous Drainage

The venous blood from the interior of the spinal cord is drained by intra-medullary radicles or internal spinal veins which join the perimedullary branches and in turn become the radicular veins emptying into the venous plexus of the intraspinal and extraspinal veins commonly called Batson's plexus. In contrast to arterial supply, the posterior spinal vein (PSV) is larger than the one or several small anterior and lateral external spinal veins. The PSV sits within or near the posterior median sulcus and extends the length of the spinal cord. It drains approximately two-thirds of the cord. In the high cervical region drainage is into the jugular veins or inferior petrosal sinus. In the cervicothoracic region drainage is into the superior intercostal veins that join the azygos system. In the dorsal region the azygos and hemiazygos veins receive the venous blood, and in the lumbar region the ascending lumbar veins join the iliac veins and inferior vena cava.

ANGIOGRAPHIC TECHNIQUE

Angiography of the spine and spinal cord was first developed in 1964 by Djindjian and Di Chiro.[4,7,8,11]

Materials

The realization of spinal angiography necessitates a classic x-ray table that ideally permits the division of the film into three parts. This is necessary because it allows a film to be obtained prior to injection of contrast material and then early and late following injection. This permits subtraction of the films for clarification of the small branches. Rapid sequence cut film units are cumbersome because of the set-up time and high numbers of films produced for each run. More recently, digital subtraction angiography units have been utilized for explorations of the spinal cord vascular supply; however, a high definition unit (1024 × 1024 matrix, 30 cm field of view) is indispensable. In general, film-based systems offer a higher degree of resolution. Occasionally, polytomography is a useful adjunct.

For spinal cord angiography a 5-F (inside diameter) sheath is placed in the femoral artery in a classic Seldinger manner. The angiographic catheter utilized is usually a 4 or 5 French with a distal hole. The distal curvature employed is variable; however, in order to seat the tip the descending portion of the catheter must usually be wedged against the opposite wall of the aorta.

Currently it is preferable to utilize nonionic contrast materials due to their decreased toxicity and diminished pain with injection. Dosages range from 2 cc for fluoroscopic testing of catheter position to 5 cc for a usual run, or occasionally 10-12 cc in cases of arteriovenous malformations or for the study of venous drainage.

The complete exploration of the vascular supply to the spinal cord may result in significantly elevated contrast loads and occasionally necessitates interrupting the examination, which can be recommenced several days later. For this reason, a serum BUN and creatinine are drawn before the examination to exclude or prepare patients with impaired renal function.

Methods

Exploration of vascular supply to the cervical spinal cord necessitates selective angiography of the following branches of the subclavian arteries: both vertebrals in the anteroposterior and lateral projection, both thyrocervical arteries, both costocervical arteries, the ascending and occasionally deep arteries, and the first intercostal branches (if separate from the costocervicals). Nonselective global subclavian arteriography by the retrograde or brachial route is reserved for young children and infants.

The study of the dorsal and lumbar spinal cord is performed by selective injection of all intercostal and lumbar arteries, the ilio-lumbar and hypogastric branches from the iliac arteries, and the middle and lateral sacral branches. Global arteriography with injection in the main distal aorta is unacceptable except in the young infant as resolution is unsatisfactory.

Occasionally the axillary approach is necessary, particularly in patients with pronounced atherosclerotic change of the femoral arteries. In this group a more rigid 6 French catheter is usually necessary to achieve torque control.

The position of the ostia of the intercostal arteries varies from one patient to another; however, their origins are paired at any given level and are in a relatively straight cephalocaudal line in any given patient. The origins of the first intercostals are very close to the first portion of the descending aorta close to the arch. It is necessary to engage these selectively and not to be content with partial visualization of these branches secondary to muscular collaterals from injection in adjacent and more inferior intercostals.

In the case of spinal arteriovenous malformations, an exhaustive examination is necessary and should include not only the more traditional selective studies but also occasionally vessels remote from the malformation as these may give blood supply. Angiotomography as well as prolonged serial filming following injection may be necessary. In vertebral body or intramedullary tumor or spinal trauma the selective examination is limited to two or three levels adjacent to the lesion.

Anesthesia

General anesthesia with endotracheal intubation is rarely necessary currently.[15] More often the examination is performed under neuroleptic anesthesia or after simple premedication with diazepam and, of course, local anesthesia at the puncture site.

Morbidity

The risks of spinal angiography are similar to those of cerebral angiography. There is the risk of dislodgement of atheromatous material into the artery being examined. There is the risk of occluding the ostium with the catheter tip, even though it is on a temporary basis. Finally, there is the risk of trauma to the artery itself from the catheterization technique. These complications are usually preventable but may occur or be recognized when there is poor collateral blood supply such as in trauma or tumor situations. Complications may occur in catheterization of the major trunks such as the artery of Adamkiewicz, with devastating consequences such as paraplegia. As in cerebral angiography, the risks diminish considerably when the angiographer has achieved technical proficiency.

The catheter should remain in the ostium only as long as necessary, specifically only for planning of the filming and during the actual filming. The catheter should then be withdrawn immediately. The advantage of appropriate shaping of the catheter such that engagement of the ostium is relatively automatic makes the use of a guide wire rarely necessary. This further reduces the risks. If these precautions are taken the patient rarely will be symptomatic during injection; however, on occasion pain and/or muscle spasm is localized to the segment injected. In such instances instillation of 1–2 ml of a solution of 10 ml of diazepam and 10 ml of normal saline usually provides immediate relief. The cause of the discomfort should be analyzed (for example, the catheter technique) and the films analyzed for the possibility of occlusion of the vessel with resultant ischemia downstream. Rarely are there permanent neurologic sequelae from the catheterization procedure. However, the need for and risks of anticoagulation should be discussed with the attending physician.

ANGIOGRAPHY OF THE NORMAL SPINAL CORD
Cervical Spinal Cord

In the AP projection the anterior spinal artery derived from the V4 segment of the vertebral artery descends to the C1 level where it continues rather vertically in the midline to the C3–C4 level where it is joined by the inconstant anastomotic branch of the ascending portion of the artery of the cervical enlargements.[7,11] The anterior meningeal branch of the vertebral artery given off just proximal to the undersurface of C2 courses obliquely toward the midline and might be confused in the AP projection but is anterior to the spinal artery in the lateral view. The anterior spinal artery frequently receives a radiculo-medullary branch

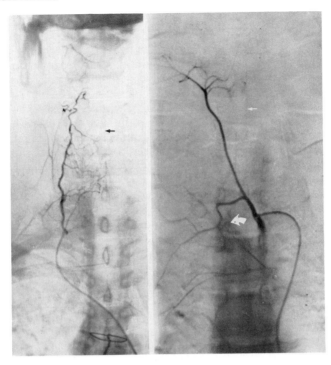

FIGURE 3. (*left*). Anterior spinal artery (arrow) with its origin from the right deep cervical artery.

FIGURE 4. (*right*). Anterior spinal artery (arrow) originating from the right T2 intercostal, posterior branch. Note also the bronchial artery branch (curved arrow).

at the C3 or C4 level from the vertebral artery given off at the C4–C5 or C5–6 level. The radiculo-medullary branches of the lower cervical cord often are given off by different branches of the subclavian arteries. The muscular branches, particularly from the ascending and deep cervical arteries, are important for their contribution to the collateral anastomotic network (Fig. 3). The much finer branches that were discussed under the anatomical section are rarely visualized during normal cervical angiography.

High Dorsal Spinal Cord

A radiculo-medullary arterial branch formed from the third, fourth, or fifth intercostal artery (usually on the left) joins the anterior spinal artery by dividing into ascending and descending branches.[3,4,7,11] The posterior spinal network is more often invisible angiographically. One can differentiate between the muscular branches that course median or paramedian from the radiculo-medullary artery by the anastomotic pattern of the former with the muscular branches of the adjacent dermatomes (Fig. 4).

Dorsal Lumbar Spinal Cord

The anterior spinal artery at this level is formed primarily by the artery of Adamkiewicz, which courses around the inferior aspect of the pedicle rising within the spinal canal toward the midline where it divides into an ascending branch and one that takes a hairpin turn, descending to join the main trunk of the anterior spinal artery.[7,10] Caudal to that region the normally straight and midline anterior spinal artery becomes sinusoidal in the region of the conus medullaris. In the lateral projection, however, it maintains a straight appearance anterior to the spinal cord (Fig. 5).

The posterior spinal artery is more often visible at this level than in the upper dorsal region. The radicular origins of these arteries form a much more acute angle of the hairpin turn than that of Adamkiewicz and its caliber is much less. In the AP view they are always paramedian in location, and in the lateral are relatively far from the posterior border of the vertebral body (Fig. 6).

The anastomotic network around the conus medullaris and the meningeal arteries more peripheral in location are normally not seen during angiography. During all intercostal injections there is visualization of a portion of the vertebral body as a stain.

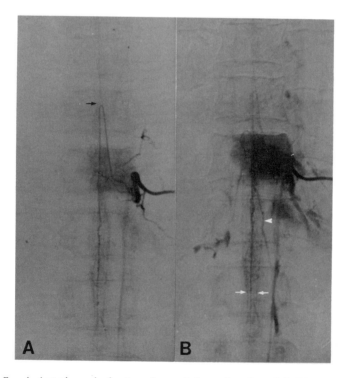

FIGURE 5. *A,* Anterior spinal artery (arrow) formation from left T11 radiculo-medullary branch. Note especially the hairpin turn of the anterior radiculo-medullary branch to anterior spinal artery. *B,* There is reflux into the posterior spinal arteries via the anastomotic loop of the conus (arrow) and visibility of the venous drainage (arrow head) on the delayed views (variation of normal). Only the ipsilateral hemivertebral body is opacified.

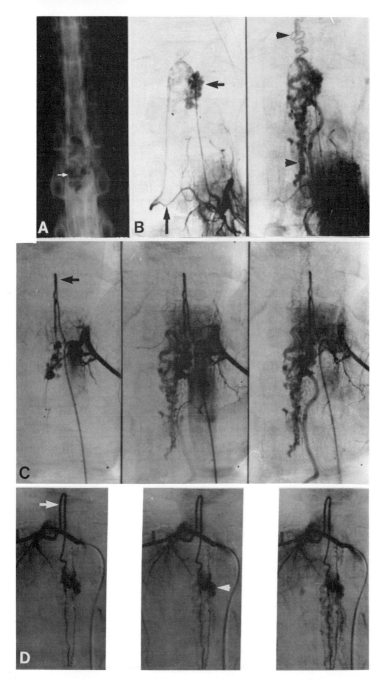

FIGURE 6. *A,* Intramedullary AVM of conus. Tomogram of dorsolumbar junction following myelogram. Note tortuous enlarged vessels (arrow). *B,* Early and late arterial phase of left L1 lumbar artery injection. Note the AVM nidus (arrow) and venous drainage (arrowheads). Also note the retrovertebral (long arrow) branch anastomosing right and left anterior radiculo-medullary arteries. *C,* Left T11 intercostal injection shows additional supply to nidus. The hairpin turn is much sharper (arrow) than that of the anterior radiculo-medullary anterior spinal supply (Fig. 3). *D,* Right T12 intercostal opacifies artery of Adamkiewicz (arrow), then anastomotic loop of conus, then posterior spinal arteries, and finally nidus (arrowhead).

THERAPEUTIC INDICATIONS
Vertebral Body Tumors

Spinal angiography permits the identification of radiculo-medullary branches before embolization by the endovascular route, surgery, or radiotherapy. The opacification of the neoplasm is therefore performed for etiologic purposes as well as for eventual treatment (Fig. 7).[8]

In hemangiomas of the vertebral body, the vertebral body shows a heterogeneous stain initially secondary to the numerous confluent channels, but these areas fill in over time, leading to rather homogeneous opacification (Fig. 8).[12] Angiography permits a better appreciation of both the intraosseous and extraosseous extension, whose dimensions were probably hinted at by prior radiographic investigation such as CT.

In contrast to hemangiomas, metastatic lesions are characterized by multiple arteriovenous fistulas and poorly circumscribed borders.

Spinal Cord and Intradural Tumors

Hemangioblastomas[13] show an angiographic picture similar to that of cerebellar hemangioblastomas, with their fine lacy globular-shaped arterial pattern and usual single draining vein. The purpose of a complete examination of the spinal cord is to define precisely the arterial supply, be it anterior spinal artery or posterior spinal artery, the exact volume of the lesion, the venous drainage,

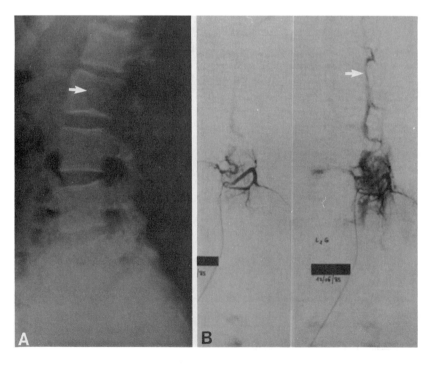

FIGURE 7. *A*, Aneurysmal bone cyst (arrow) of L2 is seen on a lateral plain film in a 15-year-old female. There is lucency of the vertebral body and pedicle with expansion of dimensions. *B*, Early and late arterial phase of left L2 lumbar arteriogram showing hypervascularization and early venous drainage (arrow).

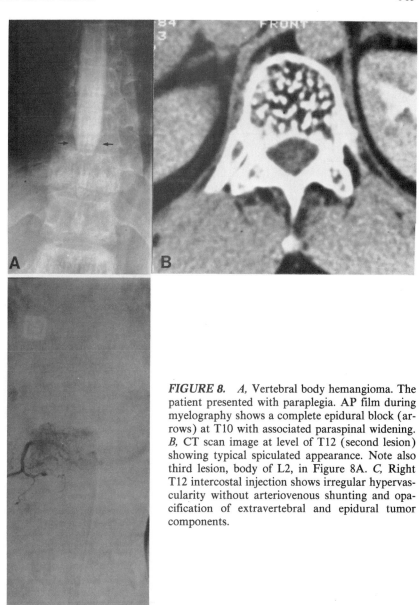

FIGURE 8. *A,* Vertebral body hemangioma. The patient presented with paraplegia. AP film during myelography shows a complete epidural block (arrows) at T10 with associated paraspinal widening. *B,* CT scan image at level of T12 (second lesion) showing typical spiculated appearance. Note also third lesion, body of L2, in Figure 8A. *C,* Right T12 intercostal injection shows irregular hypervascularity without arteriovenous shunting and opacification of extravertebral and epidural tumor components.

and as they are commonly multiple, the number (Fig. 9). In contrast to arteriovenous malformations, the border of hemangioblastomas is sharp, the stain persists for a long time, and the venous drainage appears relatively late. A complete examination includes study of the spine as well as the cerebellum to

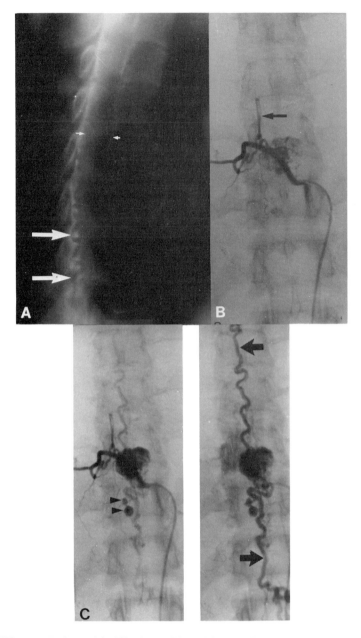

FIGURE 9. *A,* Patient with difficulty walking without a clinical level hemangioblastoma. Patient had a cerebellar hemangioblastoma removed 10 years previously. Lateral view of thoracic region during myelogram shows expansion of cord (small arrows) and dilated vessels (large arrows). *B* and *C,* Right T10 arteriography shows hypervascular mass supplied by posterior spinal artery (arrow) originating from radiculo-medullary branch. There is superior and inferior venous drainage (large arrow). Note the two additional hemangioblastomas inferiorly (arrowheads).

exclude additional unsuspected lesions, and evaluation of the visceral organs in patients with von Hippel-Lindau syndrome.

Angiographic examination of patients with intramedullary lesions visualized on myelography is important as arteriovenous malformations that may present as a mass and have draining vessels apparent on myelography have a different angiographic pattern than intramedullary glial tumors such as astrocytomas and ependymomas, which also commonly show enlarged surface vessels on myelography.[8] Angiography confirms the exact location of the tumor by demonstrating anterior and posterior spinal artery displacement; however, usually no actual tumor opacification is seen (Fig. 10).

Neuronomas show a variable angiographic pattern and their extra spinal extent is usually better demonstrated by CT or MRI. However, in the cervical region spinal angiography could be justified to define the extent of vertebral artery displacement and the radiculo-medullary branches in order to assist in surgical planning.

Arteriovenous Malformations

Arteriovenous malformations (AVMs) are characterized by arteriovenous fistulas and the absence of an observed capillary phase. An AVM may be an isolated lesion such as in cutaneous angioma or vertebral hemangioma, it may be regional such as in Klippel-Trenaunay syndrome, or diffuse as in Osler-Weber-Rendu syndrome. Spinal angiography is indispensable in the diagnostic work-up as treatment depends on the exact blood supply.[5,6,9] Without exception all AVMs fed either partially or totally by the anterior spinal artery have an intramedullary component (Figs. 6, 11, 12). In contrast if the AVM is fed exclusively by the posterior spinal artery, it will be extramedullary in location. Two distinct AVMs at the same level, one intramedullary the other extrame-

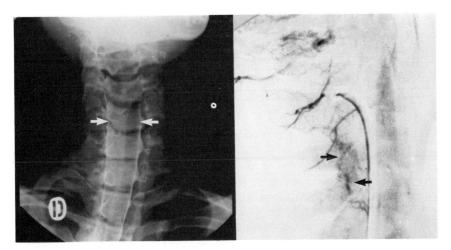

FIGURE 10. *A,* A 19-year-old with progressive proximal weakness of the lower extremities with sphincter weakness due to astrocytoma. Cervical myelogram demonstrates widening of the cervical cord (arrows). *B,* Late arterial phase vertebral artery injection lateral view shows blush and puddling of contrast between C3 and C4 (arrows).

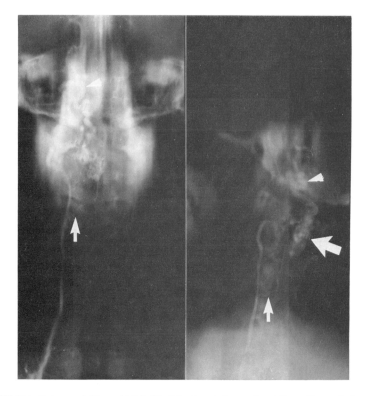

FIGURE 11.   Intramedullary AVM. Vertebral arteriography AP and lateral views show radiculo-medullary supply at C4 (arrows) to anterior spinal artery supplying a large tangle of vessels. Venous drainage (arrowheads) is superior and intracranial.

dullary, mandate a postoperative angiogram to exclude the possibility of an unrecognized small intramedullary residual.[6]

Finally, extradural or extraspinal AVMs may drain preferentially toward the intraspinal venous plexus and be responsible for myelopathy on the basis of mass effect or increased venous pressure (Fig. 13).[1,14,15]

Spinal Trauma

In severe spinal trauma with or without neurologic deficits, spinal angiography is required for an understanding of the supply to the anterior spinal artery prior to surgical stabilization by the anterior approach. In severe neurologic deficit, angiography may disclose interruption of the anterior spinal artery, which would have significant prognostic implications. Alternatively the spinal artery may be displaced anteriorly by cord swelling or hemorrhage, or may be normal in appearance and position, suggesting the possibility for improvement in neurologic status.[16,17]

Kyphosis and Scoliosis

The examination of patients destined for surgical correction of kyphosis or scoliosis permits the identification of the radiculo-medullary branches to avoid

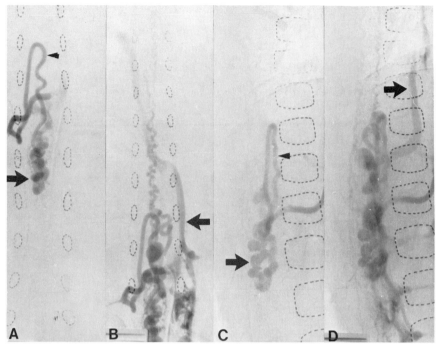

FIGURE 12. *A* and *B* are anteroposterior views. *C* and *D* are lateral views. Three-year-old child with intramedullary AVM. Right T12 injection, early and late arterial phases, show a large nidus (arrow) supplied by a dilated anterior spinal artery (arrowhead). Venous drainage is early and ventral to cord and ultimately drains into azygos system (large arrows).

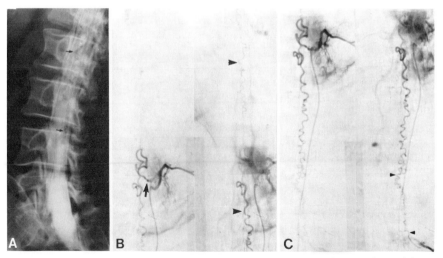

FIGURE 13. *A*, Dural AVM with medullary venous drainage in a patient with progressive paraparesis. Myelogram – oblique lumbar film shows abnormal vessels (arrows). *B* and *C*, Arteriovenous fistula (arrow) at point of penetration of dura. Venous drainage is ascending and descending (arrowheads) and is excessive.

intraoperative neurologic complications secondary to occlusion of the important primary supplying arteries.

CONCLUSION

The knowledge of spinal cord vascular anatomy is important not only to the neuroradiologist, who performs this angiography, but also to the general vascular radiologist, who is called upon to perform visceral embolizations. The consequences of inadvertent radiculo-medullary occlusion can be avoided by a thorough knowledge of the position of the ostia and collateral supply to the spinal cord.

REFERENCES

1. Castaigne P, Bories J, Brunet P, et al: Fistules artério-veineuses méningées pures à drainage veineux cortical. Rev Neurol 132:169–181, 1976.
2. Chiras J, Morvan G, Merland JJ: The angiographic appearances of the normal intercostal and lumbar arteries. Analysis and the anatomic correlation of the lateral branches. J Neuroradiol 6:169–196, 1979.
3. Crock HV, Yoshizawa H: Blood supply of the vertebral column and spinal cord in man. Berlin, Springer Verlag, 1977.
4. Di Chiro G, Wener L: Angiography of the spinal cord. J Neurosurg 39:1–29, 1973.
5. Di Chiro G, Doppman H, Ommaya AS: Selective arteriography of arteriovenous aneurysms of the spinal cord. Radiology 88:1065–1077, 1967.
6. Djindjian M, Djindjian R: Malformations vasculaires de la moelle épinière. Encycl Med Chir, Paris, 1980, Neurologie, 17067 C 10.
7. Djindjian R, Hurth M, Houdart R: Angiography of the Spinal Cord. Paris, Masson, 1970.
8. Djindjian R, Hurth M, Houdart R: Angiographie médullaire. Encycl Med Chir, Paris, 1973, Neurologie, 17032 F 10.
9. Djindjian R, Merland JJ, Djindjian M, Houdart R: Place de l'embolisation dans le traitement des malformations artério-veineuses médullaires. A propos de 38 cas. Neuroradiology 16:428–429, 1978.
10. Doppman JL, Di Chiro G: The arteria radicularis magna. Radiographic anatomy in the adult. Br J Radiol 41:40–45, 1968.
11. Doppman JL, Di Chiro G, Ommaya AR: Selective Arteriography of the Spinal Cord. St Louis, Warren H. Green, 1969.
12. Gaston A, Nguyen JP, Djindjian M, et al: Vertebral haemangioma: CT and arteriographic features in three cases. J Neuroradiol 12:21–33, 1985.
13. Hurth M, Djindjian R, Houdart R, Rey A: Hémangioblastomes intra-rachidiens. Neurochirurgie 21:1–130, 1975.
14. Kendall BE, Logue V: Spinal epidural angiomatous malformations draining into the intrathecal veins. Neuroradiology 13:181–189, 1977.
15. Merland JJ, Djindjian M, Chiras J, Djindjian R: Recent advances in spinal cord arteriography. In Post JD (ed): Radiographic Evaluation of the Spine. New York, Masson, 1980, pp. 623–645.
16. Roy Camille R, Bories J, Rousseau JM, et al: Données de l'artériographie médullaire dans le cadre des paraplégies et quadriplégies traumatiques. Chirurgie 105:154–160, 1979.
17. Theron J, Derlon JM, De Preux J: Angiography of the spinal cord after vertebral trauma. Neuroradiology 15:201–212, 1978.

BARRY M. TOM, MD
THERESA C. POWER, DO

DIAGNOSIS OF SPINAL COLUMN INFECTIONS

Reprint requests to:
Theresa C. Power, DO
Mercy Catholic Medical Center
Department of Radiology
Lansdowne Ave. and Bailey Rd.
Darby, PA 19023

Spinal inflammation is a relatively uncommon diagnosis but an important one because neglect or misdiagnosis can have catastrophic results. Prior to the advent of antibiotics, a significant number of cases were fatal.[9] Today, infections of the spine, when discovered early, are manageable with antibiotics. Modern imaging modalities such as magnetic resonance imaging (MRI), computed tomography (CT), and nuclear scintigraphy make early diagnosis possible.

DEVELOPMENT AND ANATOMY

The vertebral column arises from the mesodermal germ cell layer. At approximately the fourth week of development, mesodermal cells migrate to surround the spinal cord and primitive notochord. Each vertebral body is intersegmental in origin: the cephalic half from one sclerotome and the caudal half from the next inferior sclerotome. The intervertebral disc is composed of the annulus fibrosus and the nucleus pulposus. Mucoid degeneration of the primitive notochord gives origin to the nucleus pulposus.[34]

In the adult, the vertebral column consists of 33 vertebrae. There are seven cervical, 12 thoracic, five lumbar, five fused sacral, and three to five coccygeal vertebrae. There are four types of spinal articulations. Three are true synovial-lined diarthrodial joints. These are the facet joints, the cervical joints of Luschka, and the thoracic rib joints. The intervertebral disc is the fourth type and this is an amphiarthrodial joint.

The ligaments of the vertebral column add stability and limit excessive motion. The anterior longitudinal ligament limits excessive extension. This ligament is continuous from the axis to the sacrum. The posterior longitudinal ligament is continuous from the axis to the sacrum along the posterior aspect of the vertebral bodies and discs within the vertebral canal. This ligament limits excessive flexion. Also limiting flexion are the ligamentum flava and the supraspinous and interspinous ligaments.

Contents of the vertebral canal include the spinal cord, meninges, and the epidural space; the epidural space contains fat and a richly anastomosing plexus of veins. The meninges are composed of three cylindrical layers. From superficial to deep, they are dura mater, arachnoid, and pia mater. Potential and actual spaces exist at certain points in relation to these membranes and the spinal cord. The subdural space, between dura and arachnoid, is a potential space. These membranes are easily separated by pathologic fluids as seen with subdural hematoma or abscess. The subarachnoid space is a true space between the arachnoid and pia mater. It is filled with cerebrospinal fluid. The pia mater contains the major arteries and veins of the spinal cord. The spinal arteries arise from the vertebral vessels and receive reinforcing branches from the segmental intercostals, lumbar, and sacral arteries. Mention of the epidural venous plexus was made earlier. This internal vertebral plexus is a valveless system of veins connecting segmental veins of the thorax, abdomen, and pelvis with those of the cranial cavity.[11]

PYOGENIC VERTEBRAL OSTEOMYELITIS

Pyogenic osteomyelitis of the spine is uncommon. Between 1917 and 1934, 4% of patients with osteomyelitis had vertebral osteomyelitis.[33] A more recent study indicated an even lower incidence of 1%.

The disease has a male predominance in childhood but occurs with equal frequency in men and women in adulthood.[2,21,23] In children, the lower thoracic and lumbar spine are the most common sites of involvement. In the adult, all levels can be involved; however, the most frequently involved is the lumbar spine.[8] Digby and Kersley[13] reported that the L2–L3 level was the most frequently involved.

Approximately 66% of cases are due to *Staphylococcus aureus.*[23,47,56] Urinary tract infections and instrument usage in the genitourinary system precede a significant number of cases. Many other organisms have been reported, including *Escherichia coli, Proteus, Streptococcus, Brucella,* and *Salmonella.*

Back pain is the predominant symptom and is usually localized to the level of involvement. Fever, malaise, and weight loss are not uncommon. Children usually present with irritability, fever, and a refusal to walk. On clinical examination, decreased range of motion and muscle spasm are typical. Local tenderness is unusual. The erythrocyte sedimentation rate is universally elevated. The leukocyte count may be elevated but is variable. Positive bacterial cultures are obtained between 40 and 60% of the time.[8,32]

Radiographic changes of pyogenic osteomyelitis often are absent at the time of presentation. Later in the course of the disease, decrease in disc space, osteopenia of adjacent vertebral bodies, new bone formation, and bony fusion can be seen (Fig. 1). Plain radiographs have a sensitivity of 82%, a specificity of 57%, and an accuracy of 73%.

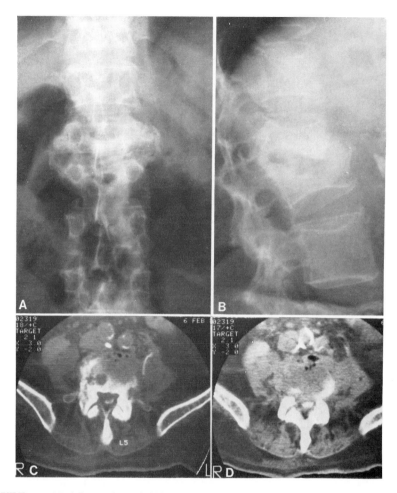

FIGURE 1. AP (*A*) and lateral (*B*) projections of thoracolumbar region in an elderly male who had undergone transurethral prostatectomy and subsequently developed staphylococcal vertebral osteomyelitis. *C* and *D,* Computed tomography following myelography in the same patient.

Bone scanning with technetium diphosphonate and MRI have enhanced early diagnosis of vertebral osteomyelitis. Technetium bone scan has a sensitivity of 90%, a specificity of 78%, and an accuracy of 86%. Combined gallium citrate and technetium bone scans have a sensitivity of 90%, a specificity of 100%, and an accuracy of 94%. MRI has a sensitivity of 96%, a specificity of 92%, and an accuracy of 94%.[41]

MRI of the spine for osteomyelitis usually consists of an initial sagittal or coronal image obtained using TE = 30 msec and TR = 0.5 sec. After identifying the abnormal areas, images using TE = 120 msec and TR = 2 to 3 sec are obtained.

The MRI findings in vertebral osteomyelitis have been described in the literature and are characteristic. On T1-weighted images (TE = 30 msec and TR = 0.5 sec), there is a confluent decrease in signal intensity from the vertebral bodies and the intervertebral disc space with an inability to discern the normal disc margins. These changes in signal intensity are probably secondary to the increased water content of the inflammatory process and ischemia. The T2 weighted images (TE = 120 msec and TR = 2 to 3 sec) show increased signal intensity of the vertebral bodies adjacent to the involved disc and abnormal configuration and signal intensity of the disc. The disc appears streaky and linear with loss of the intranuclear cleft.[42]

MRI has several advantages over nuclear scintigraphy in the detection of vertebral osteomyelitis. MRI is more accurate anatomically and provides significant anatomic information regarding the thecal sac and its contents. Involvement of the vertebral bodies, discs, and paravertebral regions is more readily appreciated. MRI is capable of differentiating infection from degenerative and neoplastic disease. Finally, signal intensity changes are not obscured by antibiotics as sometimes happens with gallium scanning.

Nuclear medicine has several advantages over MRI in the detection of vertebral osteomyelitis. Bone scan is not as sensitive as MRI to motion degradation or patient positioning. Involvement of extravertebral osseous or soft tissue structures are shown with whole body images. Gallium is more accurate in the detection of epidural abscess that does not involve bone.[42]

Antibiotic therapy of pyogenic osteomyelitis has been described in the literature.[13,52] Appropriate therapy appears to improve the resolution of the affected disc space on T1-weighted images. These changes toward normal occur anywhere from 6 to 24 weeks after the initiation of therapy.[41]

Ross and Fleming,[51] in a retrospective study of 37 cases of vertebral osteomyelitis, demonstrated several neurologic complications. These included infection of the femoral nerve, extension to the epidural space, paraparesis, paralysis, and death. Factors that increase the risk of permanent paralysis secondary to osteomyelitis are increasing age, cervical spine involvement, infection by *S. aureus,* and the presence of diabetes mellitus or rheumatoid arthritis.[16]

TUBERCULOUS SPONDYLITIS

The association of spinal deformity and paralysis with tuberculous spondylitis was first described by Pott in 1779.[46] Tuberculosis was the leading cause of death in Western society during the early 1900s.[37] Today, tuberculous spondylitis is effectively managed with chemotherapy alone in approximately 85% of cases.[15,22,39]

Lifeso et al.[35] reported 107 cases of tuberculous spondylitis. The average age of patients was 41.8 years (range, 16–75 years). The most common region of involvement was the lower thoracic and upper lumbar spine.

Diagnosis is often difficult. Bone scan is negative in 35%, gallium scan is negative in 70%, and tuberculin skin tests are negative in 14%.[35] Typical radiographic findings are irregularity of the vertebral endplates, decreased height of the disc, sclerosis, and, later, anterior wedging and or fusion (Fig. 2).[49,60] Most cases are secondary to hematogenous extent of organisms.

Differentiation between pyogenic and tuberculous osteomyelitis is often difficult. Digby and Kersley[13] listed four features of pyogenic osteomyelitis that are helpful but not diagnostically conclusive. These include the lack of significant osteoporosis, rare preservation of the disc space, and usually no large paraspinal mass, and subsequent changes that lead to healing.[13] Features more characteristic of tuberculous spondylitis are large paraspinal abscesses that are often bilateral and located caudal to the level of spondylitis, small calcifications within the abscesses, and involvement of the posterior elements.[12,35]

The MRI changes of tuberculous spondylitis are frequently similar to those seen in pyogenic osteomyelitis. Gadolinium-DTPA is a paramagnetic contrast agent helpful in demonstrating the communication of the vertebral and para-vertebral components of inflammation.[12]

Favorable results with chemotherapy alone can be achieved approximately 85% of the time. Indications for surgical intervention include neurologic impairment, spinal instability, or failure of medical management. Lifeso et al. prescribe anterior decompression and fusion as the surgical procedure of choice.[35]

INFECTION WITHIN THE SPINAL CANAL

Abscesses within the spinal canal are rare. These most commonly occur in the epidural space. Abscesses may also occur in the subdural space or they may involve the spinal cord in the intramedullary space.

Spinal Epidural Abscess

Spinal epidural abscess is an uncommon disease that occurs at a rate of about one case per year at large referral hospitals.[4,27,29,31] As with vertebral osteomyelitis, *S. aureus* is the most common causative organism. The thoracic and lumbar regions are most frequently involved.

Infection may reach the epidural space hematogenously from a distant focus, by direct extension, or by the lymphatic system. Heusner[27] reported that 75 to 80% of patients have a history of previous or concurrent infection outside the epidural space. Most commonly responsible are previous skin infections (furuncles, acne, or cellulitis). A history of trauma precedes the disease in approximately 25% of cases.[24,31] Vertebral osteomyelitis is complicated by epidural abscess in 20% of cases.

Pain is the most consistent symptom, and 90% of cases have localized tenderness. Fever, malaise, and leukocytosis are usually present. The progression of symptoms include spinal ache, root pain, symptoms of early cord impairment, and finally paralysis of cord function.[27]

Radiographs of the involved level show the changes of vertebral osteomyelitis approximately 45% of the time (Fig. 3).[4,29] With normal radiographs and a high clinical suspicion, myelography is the definitive diagnostic test. Myelography nearly always shows an epidural mass (Fig. 4). Computed tomography after myelography further enhances the diagnosis (Fig. 5).

The major consideration of differential diagnosis is acute transverse myelitis. This is a disease of uncertain etiology. It occurs 8 to 20 times more frequently than epidural abscess.[1] It is characterized by the onset of muscle weakness, loss of pain and temperature sensation, and rapid progression (usually within 24 to 48 hours) to maximum neurologic deficit.[36] Absence of back pain and reaching maximum neurologic deficit in less than 72 hours favors the diagnosis of acute transverse myelitis. Factors favoring epidural abscess include abnormal myelogram, recent bacterial infection, especially staphylococcal, and radiographic evidence of vertebral osteomyelitis.[1] Subdural empyema and meningitis are other diagnostic considerations; neither of these typically shows local tenderness.

Spinal Subdural Empyema

Spinal subdural empyema is uncommon, with only 10 reported cases in the literature. Several features are common to most cases. These include a history

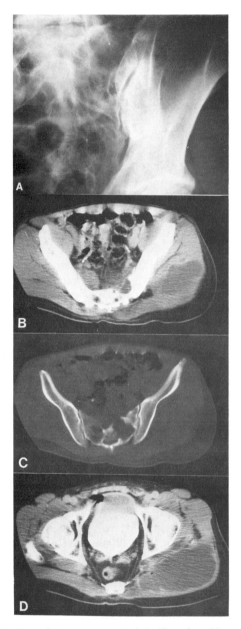

FIGURE 2. *A,* Plain film of the sacrum and right ilium in a 50-year-old male with pain in the lower back and left buttock. The film demonstrates subtle bony demineralization of the sacrum. *B–D,* Computed tomography shows a destructive process involving the left sacrum with a large associated gluteal abscess.

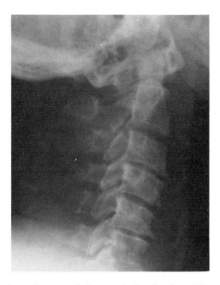

FIGURE 3. A single lateral view of the cervical spine in a 50-year-old black male with a long history of intravenous drug abuse. Changes consistent with vertebral osteomyelitis are seen at the C6–C7 level.

of previous or concurrent bacterial infection, absence of vertebral tenderness, slowly evolving neurologic deficit, and cerebrospinal fluid and myelographic evidence of parameningeal inflammation.[19]

Clinically, spinal subdural empyema mimics epidural abscess except for the lack of localized tenderness. *Staphylococcus aureus* is the most common causative agent. The cerebrospinal fluid is always abnormal with elevated protein, decreased glucose levels, and pleocytosis.

The differential diagnosis includes spinal epidural abscess and acute transverse myelitis. Rapidly evolving neurologic deficit favors acute transverse myelitis. Previous or concurrent infection favors epidural and subdural abscess and these are differentiated at surgery.

Spinal Cord Abscess

Spinal cord abscess is less common than either epidural or subdural abscess. Only 54 cases have been reported since Hart[26] reported the first case in 1830. Review of the literature indicates that spinal cord abscess is a disease of childhood with 40% of cases occurring during the first two decades of life, with most (27%) before age 10.[14]

The thoracic cord is most commonly involved and *S. aureus* is the most common causative organism. Most cases are secondary to metastatic spread from remote infections. Infected dermal sinuses, paravertebral infection, lumbar puncture, surgical intervention, and trauma may also lead to spinal cord abscess.[38]

Patients with spinal cord abscess consistently have pain in the spine and dysesthesia.[3,17,18,43,44,50,59] The acute presentation is partial or complete transverse myelitis preceded by neck or back pain and urinary incontinence. Chronic abscess presents similar to intramedullary tumor.[40] The outcome is favorable using both antibiotics and surgical intervention.

INFLAMMATION OF THE MENINGES
Bacterial Meningitis

Bacterial meningitis has an incidence of 5 to 10 cases per 100,000 persons per year. Incidence is highest during the first month of life, occurring in 1.3 per 10,000 full-term births, and in 24 per 10,000 premature births.[6]

Hemophilus influenzae, Neisseria meningitidis, and *Streptococcus pneumoniae* account for 80% of all cases of bacterial meningitis.[10] *Hemophilus influenzae* accounts for approximately half of the cases. Meningitis secondary to this organism occurs primarily under the age of 5 years with approximately 85%

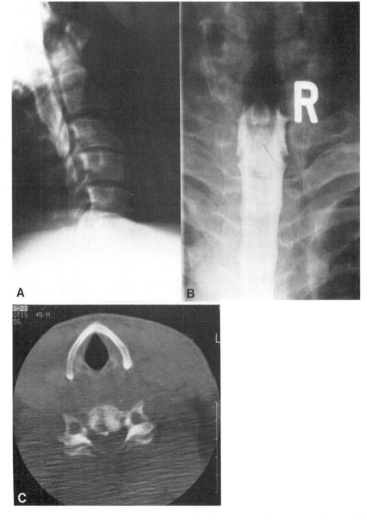

FIGURE 4. *A* and *B*, Myelography via cervical puncture shows complete block at the C4–C5 level. Lumbar myelography demonstrates block at the C7–T1 level. *C,* Computed tomography after myelography through the C6 level shows complete block as well as changes in the adjacent vertebral body. At surgery, epidural abscess was demonstrated.

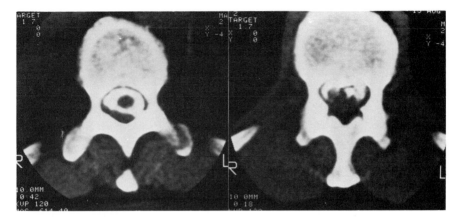

FIGURE 5. A 70-year-old white male presented with acute radicular pain of the lower extremity. Physical examination was consistent with acute disc herniation. Also noted was a carbuncle on the patient's back. Post-myelography computed tomography reveals posterior epidural abscess, which was positive for staphylococcus at surgery.

occurring between 1 month and 2 years. *Neisseria meningitidis* accounts for 25% of cases and occurs primarily during the first year of life. *Streptococcus pneumoniae* accounts for 10–15% of cases and occurs in children younger than 2 years. There is an increased risk for pneumococcal infection, including pneumococcal meningitis, with splenic dysfunction (sickle cell disease), Hodgkin's disease, multiple myeloma, alcoholism, and renal or bone marrow transplants.[7] Recurrent pneumococcal meningitis has been reported in patients with cerebrospinal fluid leaks secondary to trauma or neurosurgical procedures.[25]

Several clinical and laboratory findings are common to most cases of bacterial meningitis. Fever and peripheral leukocytosis are almost always present. The classic signs of meningeal irritation, including stiffness of the neck and back, Hoyne's sign, and Brudzinski's and Kernig's signs, are usually present. However, these signs frequently are absent in infants and the elderly. Often a bulging fontanelle is the only finding with infants.[61]

Cerebrospinal fluid examination is the primary diagnostic procedure. Findings with bacterial meningitis include increased white cells with polymorphonuclear leukocyte predominance, increased protein, and decreased glucose levels. Early in bacterial meningitis the glucose level may be normal. It is important to note that early in aseptic meningitis there may be a polymorphonuclear leukocyte predominance; however, this usually converts to mononuclear predominance later in the course of the disease. Early diagnosis and treatment is essential. Probably the most critical factor in determining prognosis is the timing of therapy.

Neonatal bacterial meningitis occurs in the first few days of life. Maternal complications such as premature rupture of membranes, premature labor, and peripartum maternal infection often accompany neonatal meningitis. *Escherichia coli* and group B *Streptococcus* are the most frequent causative organisms. The cerebrospinal fluid findings are often equivocal. Blood cultures show bacteremia in approximately one fourth of cases. As with meningitis later in life, early diagnosis and treatment are essential.

Viral Meningitis

Viral meningitis is the most common type of aseptic meningitis. Aseptic meningitis may also be secondary to *Mycoplasma pneumoniae, Mycobacteria,* fungi, and *Toxoplasmosis.*

Findings in the cerebrospinal fluid in viral meningitis include mononuclear pleocytosis (20% to 70% have polymorphonuclear leukocyte predominance early on), variable increase in protein, normal glucose, and no evidence of organisms. The clinical findings are nonspecific. Headache, fever, nausea, vomiting, malaise, and nuchal rigidity are some of the findings. Infants frequently only have fever and irritability.

The most commonly identified causative virus is the enterovirus.[20,45] Enterovirus (poliovirus, coxsackievirus, and echovirus) is spread by the fecal-oral route and is seen most often in individuals with poor personal hygiene. Enterovirus infections peak in the summer.

Arachnoiditis (Noninfectious Meningitis)

Arachnoiditis is a misnomer. In reality, inflammation involves all three meningeal layers (dura, arachnoid, and pia). Review of the literature shows several causative factors. Spinal anesthesia, myelographic contrast agents (especially pantopaque and ionic water soluble agents), neoplasm, meningitis (pyogenic, syphilitic, tuberculous), and traumatic and nontraumatic hemorrhage are factors.[48] Blood and contrast agents appear to be synergistic in the production of arachnoiditis.[5,28]

The changes seen radiographically in arachnoiditis range from mild to severe. Nerve root sleeve blunting and small lateral defects are seen with mild arachnoiditis. Complete obliteration of the arachnoid space can be seen in severe cases.[30,53,57] MRI shows heterogeneous signal intensity from the thecal sac secondary to arachnoiditis.

A significant number of cases of arachnoiditis are clinically asymptomatic. Suolanen[57] showed that neurologic symptoms after myelography with the water-soluble agent Conturex were rare despite the high frequency of arachnoiditis. The newer water-soluble, non-ionic myelographic contrast agents have almost completely eliminated arachnoiditis as a complication after myelography.[54,55]

REFERENCES

1. Altrocchi PH: Acute spinal epidural abscess vs. acute transverse myelopathy. Arch Neurol 9:17, 1963.
2. Ambrose GB, Alpert M, Neer CS: Vertebral osteomyelitis—a diagnostic problem. JAMA 197:101, 1966.
3. Artz, PK: Abscess within the spinal cord: Review of literature and report of 3 cases. Arch Neurol Psychiatry 51:533–543, 1944.
4. Baker, AS, Ojemann RG, Swartz MN, et al: Spinal epidural abscess. N Engl J Med 293:463, 1975.
5. Bergeron UT, Rumbaugh CL, Fang H, et al: Experimental Pantopaque arachnoiditis in the monkey. Radiology 99:95–101, 1971.
6. Berman PH, Banker BQ: Neonatal meningitis. Pediatrics 38:6, 1966.
7. Bolan G, Barza M: Acute bacterial meningitis in children and adults. Med Clin North Am 69:231–241, 1985.
8. Bonfiglio M, Lange TA, Kim YM: Pyogenic vertebral osteomyelitis. Clin Orthop 96:234, 1973.
9. Butler GCB, Bhusger IN, Perry KMA: Staphylococcal osteomyelitis of the spine. Lancet 1:480–481, 1941.
10. Centers for Disease Control: Bacterial meningitis and meningococcemia—U.S. MMWR 28:277, 1979.

11. Clemente C: Anatomy, A Regional Atlas of the Human Body, 2nd ed. Baltimore, Urban & Schwarzenberg, 1981, pp 463–506.
12. de Roos A, van Persijn van Meerlen EL, Bloem JL, Bluemm RG: MRI of tuberculous spondylitis. AJR 146:79–82, 1986.
13. Digby JM, Kersley JB: Pyogenic non-tuberculous spinal infection. Analysis of thirty cases. J Bone Joint Surg 61B(1):47–55, 1979.
14. Ditullio MV: Intramedullary spinal abscess: A case report with a review of 53 previously described cases. Surg Neurol 7:351–354, 1977.
15. Editorial: Tuberculosis of the spine. Med J 4:613–614, 1974.
16. Eismont FJ, Bohlman HH, Soni PL, et al: Pyogenic and fungal vertebral osteomyelitis with paralysis. J Bone Joint Surg 65A:19–29, 1983.
17. El Gindi S, Fairburn B: Intramedullary spinal abscess as complication of congenital dermal sinus. J Neurosurg 30:494–497, 1969.
18. Foley J: Intramedullary abscess of the spinal cord. Lancet 2:193–195, 1949.
19. Fraser RA, Ratzan K, Wolpert SM, Weinstein L: Spinal subdural empyema. Arch Neurol 28:235–238, 1973.
20. Galko NV, Vashukova SS, Dadiomova MA et al: Etiology of sporadic aseptic meningitis in children in the Leningrad area. Sçand J Infect Dis 11:173–174, 1979.
21. Garcia A Jr, Grantham SA: Hematogenous vertebral osteomyelitis. J Bone Joint Surg 42A:429, 1960.
22. Griffiths DL: The treatment of tuberculosis of bone and joint. J Trop Med Hyg 72:559–563, 1978.
23. Griffiths HED, Jones DM: Pyogenic infection of the spine. J Bone Joint Surg 53B:383, 1971.
24. Hancock DO: A study of 49 patients with acute spinal epidural abscess. Paraplegia 10:285, 1973.
25. Hand WL, Sanford JP: Posttraumatic bacterial meningitis. Ann Intern Med 72:869, 1970.
26. Hart J: A case of encysted abscess in the centre of the spinal cord. Dublin Hosp Rep 5:522–524, 1830.
27. Heusner AP: Nontuberculous spinal epidural infections. N Engl J Med 239:845, 1948.
28. Howland WJ, Curry JL: Experimental studies of Pantopaque arachnoiditis. Radiology 87:253–261, 1966.
29. Hulme A, Dott NM: Spinal epidural abscess. Br Med J 1:64, 1954.
30. Hurteau E, Baird WC, Sinclair E: Arachnoiditis following the use of iodonized oil. J Bone Joint Surg 36A:393–400, 1954.
31. Kaufman DM, Kaplan JG, Litman N: Infectious agents in spinal epidural abscesses. Neurology 30:844, 1980.
32. King DM, Mayo KM: Infective lesions of the vertebral column. Clin Orthop 96:248, 1973.
33. Kulowski J: Pyogenic osteomyelitis of the spine. J Bone Joint Surg 18:343, 1936.
34. Langman J: Medical Embryology, 4th ed. Baltimore, Williams & Wilkins, 1981, pp 123–137.
35. Lifeso RM, Weaver P, Harder EH: Tuberculous spondylitis in adults. J Bone Joint Surg 67A(9):1405–1412, 1985.
36. Lipton HL, Teasdale RD: Acute transverse myelopathy in adults. Arch Neurol 28:252, 1973.
37. Martin NS: Tuberculosis of the spine. A study of the results of treatment during the last twenty-five years. J Bone Joint Surg 52B(4):613–628, 1970.
38. McGeachie RE, Ford WJ, Nelson MJ, et al: Neuroradiology case of the day. AJR 148:1053–1058, 1987.
39. Medical Research Council Working Party on Tuberculosis of the Spine—First Report: A controlled trial of ambulant out-patient treatment and in-patient rest in bed in the management of tuberculosis of the spine in young Korean patients on standard chemotherapy. A study in Masan, Korea. J Bone Joint Surg 55B:678–697, 1973.
40. Menezes AH, Graf CJ, Perret GE: Spinal cord abscess: A review. Surg Neurol 8:461–467, 1977.
41. Modic MT, Feiglin DH, Piraino DW: Vertebral osteomyelitis: Assessment using MR. Radiology 157:157–166, 1985.
42. Modic MT, Pflanze W, Feiglin DH: Magnetic resonance imaging of musculoskeletal infections. Rad Clin North Am 24:247–258, 1986.
43. Nothnagel H: Ueber Ruckenmarksabscess. Wein Med Lb 7:288–289, 1884.
44. Parker RL, Collins GH: Intramedullary abscess of the brainstem and spinal cord. South Med J 63:495–497, 1976.
45. Ponka A, Petterson T: The incidence and aetiology of central nervous system infections in Helsinki in 1980. Acta Neurol Scand 66:529–535, 1982.
46. Pott P: Remarks on that kind of palsy of the lower limb, which is frequently found to accompany a curvature of the spine, and is supposed to be caused by it. Together with its method of cure. Med Classic 1(4):281–297, 1936.

47. Puig Guri J: Pyogenic osteomyelitis of the spine: Differential diagnosis through clinical and roentgenographic observations. J Bone Joint Surg 28:29, 1946.
48. Quencer RM, Tenner M, Rothman L: The postoperative myelogram. Radiology 123:667–679, 1977.
49. Resnick D, Niwayama G: Osteomyelitis, septic arthritis, and soft tissue infection: the organisms. In Diagnosis of Bone and Joint Disorders. Philadelphia, W. B. Saunders, 1981, pp 2167–2170.
50. Rifaat M, El Shafei M, et al: Intramedullary spinal abscess following spinal puncture. Neurosurgery 38:366–367, 1973.
51. Ross PM, Fleming JL: Vertebral body osteomyelitis spectrum and natural history: A retrospective analysis of 37 cases. Clin Orthop 118:190, 1976.
52. Sapico FL, Mongomerie JZ: Pyogenic vertebral osteomyelitis: Report of nine cases and review of the literature. Rev Infect Dis 1:754–776, 1979.
53. Seamen WB, Marder SN, Rosenbaum SE: The myelographic appearance of adhesive spinal arachnoiditis. J Neurosurg 10:145–153, 1953.
54. Skalpe IO, Amundsen P: Lumbar radiculopathy with metrizamide. A non-ionic water soluble contrast medium. Radiology 115:91–95, 1975.
55. Skalpe IO, Amundsen P: Thoracic and cervical myelography with metrizamide. Clinical experiences with a water-soluble non-ionic contrast medium. Radiology 116:101–106, 1975.
56. Stone DB, Bonfiglio M: Pyogenic vertebral osteomyelitis. Arch Intern Med 112:491, 1963.
57. Suolanen J: Adhesive arachnoiditis following myelography with various water soluble contrast media. Neuroradiol 9:78–83, 1975.
58. Teng P, Papatheodonic C: Myelographic findings in adhesive spinal arachnoiditis (with a brief surgical note). Br J Radiol 40:201–208, 1967.
59. Turner W, Collier J: Intramedullary abscess of spinal cord. Brain 27:199–208, 1904.
60. Weaver P, Lifeso RM: The radiologic diagnosis of tuberculosis of the adult spine. Skeletal Radiol 12:178–186, 1984.
61. Weinstein L: Bacterial meningitis: Specific etiologic diagnosis on the basis of distinctive epidemiologic, pathogenic, and clinical features. Med Clin North Am 69:219–229, 1985.

BARRY JEFFRIES, MD

FACET STEROID INJECTIONS

From the Department of Radiology
Georgia Baptist Hospital, Atlanta,
Georgia

Reprint requests to:
Barry Jeffries, MD
Department of Radiology
Georgia Baptist Hospital
300 Boulevard, NE
Atlanta, GA 30312

That the lumbar facet joints could be a source of pain was first suggested by Goldthwait in 1911 and reinforced by Putti in 1927.[7] The term "facet syndrome" was first used by Ghormley in 1933. He pointed out that many of the aches and pains known as backache or true joint pain represented the same type of joint pain seen in arthritis of other synovial joints.[1,7] Badgeley (1941) stressed the importance of the facets in low back and leg pain, feeling that 80% of low back pain and sciatica were due to referred pain and not direct nerve irritation.[7] In 1934, Mixter and Barr promoted the concept of the rupture of the intervertebral disc as the etiology of low back and leg pain. In 1956, Pederson returned attention to the facet joint as a source of pain. Hirsch (1963) confirmed this by injection of 10% normal saline in the region of the facet joints with production of pain in the back and upper thigh.[7] Mooney and Robertson found in 100 patients treated with injections of the facet joints that 62% had complete relief immediately after injection and 52% had at least partial relief 6 months after the block. These findings suggested that the lumbar disc is not the exclusive source of chronic low back pain and sciatica; and that structural, degenerative, or inflammatory disease of the facet joints may represent a major cause of low back pain with or without sciatic radiation.[1] They also indicated that objective abnormalities, such as altered deep tendon reflexes, inhibited straight-leg raising, and abnormal EMG, which are associated with lumbar disc disease, can be caused by facet arthropathy, as these objective findings returned to normal after facet injections. The specific pathophysiologic reason for these changes is not indicated by the improvement seen after facet injection.[1]

ANATOMY

Adjacent vertebral bodies are attached by the intervertebral disc anteriorly and by the apophyseal (facet) joints posterolaterally. The facet joints are formed by the superior and inferior articular processes of successive vertebrae. The facet joints are true synovial joints with hyaline cartilage surfaces and a joint space enclosed by a fibrous capsule lined with synovial membrane. These joints are oriented with varying degrees of obliquity to the sagittal plane, the degree of obliquity often varying from side to side. The capsule of the facet joint blends with the ligamentum flavum on its medial and superior aspects, which takes the place of a true joint capsule. The ligament is relatively loosely attached. The outer portions of the ligamentum flavum may prevent the capsule from being nipped between the two articular surfaces during movement and from protrusion into the intervertebral canal. The outer aspect of the articulation is covered by a fibrous layer. Because these joints move by flexion, extension, and rotation, the capsule is located behind the borders of the articular surfaces and forms recesses around them. In particular, there are large recesses covering the extremities of the apophyses. The inferior recess is always substantially larger than the other ones. The synovial lining is made up of villi that may vary in size, shape, and appearance and which contain a rich supply of blood vessels.[2,7]

Bradley (1974), and Edgar and Ghadially (1976) emphasized that the medial divisions of the posterior primary rami of segmental nerves enter the posterior compartment of the back via an osseofibrous foramen lying immediately adjacent to bone beside the facet joint rather than more laterally through or around the intertransverse ligament as inferred by Rees (1971).[4] This osseofibrous foramen is formed by the mammilloaccessory ligament, which may be ossified, connecting a small prominence on the dorsolateral surface of the superior articular process called a mammillary process with a second bony prominence called the accessory process arising from the dorsal surface of the transverse process near its junction with the superior articular process. After the medial branch of the posterior primary ramus passes through this tunnel, it gives off three branches: a proximal branch that hugs the bone, hooks on the articular process, and innervates the facet; a medial descending branch that passes medially and downward to innervate the superior and medial aspects of the capsule one level lower as well as muscular and cutaneous branches; and an ascending branch that arises from the mixed spinal nerve just anterior to the intertransverse fascia and ascends through the soft tissues to the posterior aspect of the facet above. As a result, each medial branch supplies at least three ipsilateral facet joints. No contralateral supply has been demonstrated.[4,7]

PATHOPHYSIOLOGY

The facet joints, being synovial joints, have the same types of degenerative changes encountered by larger synovial joints. However, noticeable radiographic changes are not seen in the early phase. In a study by Carrera et al. (1980) of 100 patients, CT scans showed arthropathy in many patients who had normal plain films. The nonsensitivity of plain films for detection of facet arthropathy as the cause of back pain is further supported by the work of Putti (1927), and Putti and Logroscino (1938), who found evidence of facet osteoarthritis in a series of 75 cadavers aged 40 or more.[8]

Intervertebral disc herniation has been associated with characteristic signs in the lower limb that permit accurate diagnosis and are correlated with a probable good surgical result. However, Mooney and Robertson (1976) showed that some of the signs usually associated with lumbar disc herniation, and therefore with anterior ramus compression, could be caused by pathologic changes in the facet joints. In their series, volunteers with back pain were given saline injections into their lower lumbar facet joints. Some of the volunteers developed diminution of straight-leg raising and even absence of ankle jerks. This work indicated that these effects were due to painful stimuli arising in the capsules of the facet joints and mediated by the posterior primary rami. They concluded that the only reliable neurologic signs of anterior ramus dysfunction are specific sensory or motor loss.[8]

In a middle-aged patient with chronic low back pain not radiating below the knee and with no radiologic signs of lumbar spondylosis, the principal source of pain may be difficult to determine. Several authors contend that the posterior spinal joints are largely responsible for the symptoms in this patient (Goldthwait, 1911; Ghormley, 1933; Badgley, 1941; Sinclair et al., 1948; Lewin, Moffett, and Viidik, 1962; Hockaday and Whitty, 1967; Mooney and Robertson, 1976).[8] Several mechanisms could explain the role of these articulations in lumbosciatic pain: the articular capsule is richly innervated; the medial aspect of the joint is in contact with the intervertebral foramen and, hence, with the lumbar nerve root; and the posterior ramus of the spinal nerve passes in close proximity to the lateral border of the capsule.[2] With disc degeneration, it seems logical that associated distortion of the disc height and alignment will affect the associated facet joints. As the movements between the spinal segments become uneven, excessive, and irregular, this will cause dysfunction in the facet joints with subsequent degenerative changes.[4] The poor localization of pain secondary to facet arthropathy is explained by the pattern of sensory innervation of these joints. Each joint has a "multi-level" sensory supply: by a branch of the medial division of the posterior primary ramus at its own level; by a descending branch of the medial division from the level above; and by an ascending branch from the mixed spinal nerve.[4,7]

HISTORICAL REVIEW

As the pain associated with facet arthropathy is mediated by triple innervation, early attempts used surgical and later chemical means to destroy the nerves. Rees developed a procedure of bilateral subcutaneous rhizolysis in 1971, claiming a 99.8% success rate for 2000 operations. Subsequent studies, however, have questioned the validity of his results. Shealy began to use this method, but abandoned it due to a 6% significant hematoma rate. He then turned to a temperature-controlled, radio-frequency cautery technique for denervating the facet joints. Other studies of the surgical anatomy of the facet joint seriously question whether or not a true denervation was carried out. In 1979, Bogduk and Long refined Shealy's technique, attempting to denervate selectively the medial branch of the dorsal ramus. Selby attempted denervation by injecting 10% phenol and glycerine. Direct open surgical rhizotomy has also been done. A recent controlled, double-blind study of radio-frequency rhizolysis in the management of low-back pain indicates that it did not alter the natural cause of backache or referred pain to the leg. More recent treatments have leaned toward the use of steroids.[7]

Facet joint injections with steroids and lidocaine have been used as a diagnostic and therapeutic modality. Arthrography of facet joints has been used to study patterns of referred pain. Mooney achieved long-term relief in 20% of patients and partial relief in 33% after facet injections. Park studied 100 patients with back or radicular leg pain clinically indistinguishable from the disc syndrome and found that patterns of referred pain from the facet joints could be induced in the low back, buttock, or leg by facet arthrography and could be reversed by injecting lidocaine. By injecting these joints with steroids, long-term relief occurred in 20% and partial relief in 30%.[7] Carrera (1980) used facet injections to achieve long-term relief in 30% of patients after injections of steroids and local anaesthetic. Destouet et al. (1982) achieved long-term relief in 20% of 54 patients.[8] Selby did 100 consecutive facet joint injections; 45% of the patients had no response, 26% had positive response with permanent relief, and 29% had short-term relief of which 22 were reinjected. Twelve of these last patients underwent unilateral facet desensitization with phenol with good relief.[7]

SIGNS AND SYMPTOMS

Low-back, buttock, or leg pain is a nonspecific finding that can originate in areas other than the facet joints. However, facet arthropathy can be responsible for many of the symptoms of spine pain, including sciatica. The back pain associated with leg pain and paresthesias of herniated discs may be facetogenic in nature. Symptoms of a classic facet syndrome are: hip and buttock pain; cramping leg pain, primarily above the knee; low-back stiffness, especially in the morning or with inactivity; and absence of paresthesias. The signs of a classic facet syndrome are: local paralumbar tenderness; pain on spine hyperextension; absence of neurologic deficit; absence of signs of nerve root tension; and hip, buttock, or back pain on straight leg raising. Theoretically, any abnormality of the facet joint such as inflammation, segmental instability, or degenerative arthritis can cause a facet type of syndrome. Symptoms of lumbar disc protrusion often may be similar to those of facet arthropathy, as a protruding disc may cause facet synovitis.[7]

The specific mechanism of pain production is uncertain. The facet joints are capable of various gliding motions, and their articular surfaces are not in perfect apposition. Synovial villi that are richly innervated and vascularized have been reported between the articulating surfaces. Pinching or crushing of these villi, which become hypertrophied in degenerative disease during motion, may be one source of pain. The overlapping segmental nerve supply to the facet joints helps to explain why the distribution of back and leg pain is not specific for a particular facet level. The lack of nerve supply crossing the midline to innervate contralateral facets at a given level explains the frequent unilateral nature of symptoms.[1]

Mooney and Robertson reported that the L4–5 and L5–S1 facets are frequently involved in back pain that radiates down the back of the leg, and that the L2–3 and L3–4 facets seem to be associated with pain on the side of the leg and in the area of the greater trochanter.[1] In a provocative study of facet pain referral patterns, McCall et al. found that provocative stimulation with saline of the L1–2 and L4–5 facets revealed a considerable area of common pain referral for a given site of stimulus, but with individual variation in the extent of the referral. Contrary to expectation, referral of pain to the upper groin was not a specific feature of the upper lumbar spine stimulus, but was common from the lower lumbar spine. Significant leg pain was not elicited. The presence of overlap of pain referral from the widely separated level of L1–2 and L4–5 indicates a lack of clear segmental innervation.[10] In general, there was consistency of referral to the flank region from the upper lumbar spine and to the buttocks from L4–5. There was, however, individual variation in the extent of the referral, with less uniformity at the lower level. Overlap of induced pain was experienced by most subjects over the iliac crest posteriorly and the upper groin in spite of injections four segments apart. Pain around the hernial orifices was common from the L4–5 level, but was present in only one patient from L1–2. Pain referral to the thigh occurred, but in no instance extended beyond the knee. Pain never occurred on the contralateral side of the body. There was also little difference between the distribution of referred pain from intraarticular or pericapsular injections.[10]

As mentioned earlier, the apophyseal joints are supplied by the medial branch of the corresponding posterior primary ramus, which also supplies the level below. The lumbodorsal fascia is also supplied by a continuation of the branches from the posterior primary ramus to the deep underlying sacrospinalis muscle, and overlap is present. The freely ending plexiform arrangement of the unmyelinated nerve fibers ramify in the fibrous capsule of the synovial apophyseal joints and the longitudinal flaval and interspinous ligaments. There is an absence of nerve endings in the articular cartilage and synovium. In view of this interrelation of the distribution of the nerve fibers of the posterior rami, it is not surprising that there is similarity in pain referral from intraarticular and pericapsular sources.[10]

THERAPEUTIC RESULTS

Several studies evaluating the efficacy of intraarticular injection of steroids for relief of facet induced pain have been performed. A group of 25 patients with their first significant attack of low-back or leg pain were evaluated. The facet near the maximum area of tenderness was injected with 0.5 mL of Sensorcaine after 0.2 mL of contrast for needle position confirmation. A facet joint was also injected at random. Patients were identified as responders and nonresponders. Six responders had some relief of pain from the random injection, but not the nonresponders. The responders were younger and had histories of acute onset of pain usually associated with movement, such as bending or twisting, exacerbated by sitting and relieved by walking. Nonresponders tended to have an insidious onset of pain, relieved by sitting and increased by walking. Responders had pain in the back and thigh, whereas nonresponders had pain in the back and lower leg. It was suggested that responders had a mechanical origin to their pain, probably originating in the facet joints. The mechanism of pain in the nonresponders was less clear. Two patients had neurologic signs and filling defects on myelography. The remainder may have had pain originating from a nerve root of from other possible sources in the low back.[3,6]

Lewinnek and Warfield determined that a form of restlessness they termed time-dependent positional distress and back pain great enough to wake the patient at night correlated positively with a lasting result after facet injection. In their study, all of the responders showed radiographic changes in the facet joints; they assumed that in some of the responders the facet joints would not yet have developed sclerosis or osteophytes. They concluded that x-rays must be interpreted with care in patients with recent onset of pain, for the studies may be negative. Care must also be taken with positive studies in patients who have no tenderness; the results of their study apply only to patients with all three findings of pain, tenderness, and radiographic changes.[6]

In other series, initial response rates to steroid injection of the facet joints ranged from 93% to 56%. Lasting responses (in follow-up of 6 months or more) ranged from 10% to 56% if both excellent and partial relief of pain was included.[5,6,8,11] The presence or absence of radiographic changes involving the facet joints appears to have some prognostic value, although this finding was not supported by all studies. In one series, 14 of 18 patients for whom CT or plain film studies of the lumbar area were available had narrowing of the joint cartilage space, sclerosis of the subchondral bone, or enlargement of the facet by osteophytes, leading to a diagnosis of degenerative joint disease. Of these 14 patients, 13 (93%) had an initial response and of the 12 patients followed for periods greater than three months, 5 (42%) had a lasting response. One patient had questionable changes. He had an initial good response, but pain later recurred. Of the remaining three patients with normal facets seen radiographically, there was no response to the facet injection.[6] A different study indicated that the presence or absence of structural damage on plain x-ray or CT studies was not a useful predictor of clinical outcome of facet joint steroid injections.[5]

Other factors relating to the efficacy of facet joint injections have been studied. In some studies, those patients more likely to respond to facet joint injections were younger and had relatively acute onset of pain.[3] A different study found that age and duration of symptoms were not useful predictors of outcome.[5] Involvement in litigation was a negative predictor of outcome in one study,[5] but in a different study of workmen's compensation cases, motor vehicle accident victims with pending litigation, and patients after discectomy, 52% of patients receiving facet joint injections obtained fair to excellent responses. Of those patients who received no benefit from the injections, one had vascular problems, four had spinal stenosis, three showed central disc herniation, three showed arachnoiditis, and 11 were diagnosed as having a compensation neurosis. The remaining 22 patients did not return for follow-up.[7]

Evaluation of the placement of the steroids themselves, either intraarticular or extraarticular, indicates a statistically greater probability of therapeutic response if the injection is intraarticular.[8]

In an additional study, 62 patients had 125 facet joint arthrographic examinations for complaints reminiscent of the "facet syndrome" emphasized by Mooney and Robertson in 1976. Eleven patients had spondylolysis at the lumbar level. During arthrography, 2 to 4 mL of Telebrix was injected. In 9 of 11 patients with spondylolysis, the contrast material not only opacified the injected facet joint, but also extended into the adjacent facet joint through a channel in the area of the defect. In one of the 11, the contrast extended only into a diverticular cavity in the area of spondylolysis and did not opacify the adjacent facet. One patient had no extension of contrast into the defect. In one patient with bilateral spondylolysis of L5, the contrast material injected into the left L5–S1 facet joint extended not only into the ipsilateral area of spondylolysis and the adjacent L4–5 facet, but also into the contralateral L4–5 and L5–S1 facet joints. It crossed the midline via an irregular paralaminar channel joining both areas of spondylolysis. In patients with spondylolysis, larger amounts of contrast were required to distend the facet joints and there was diffusion of contrast into the adjacent soft tissues, usually from the inferior joint recess.[9]

Communication between diseased facet joints was seen only in patients with spondylolysis. Because spondylolysis probably represents a stress lesion, bony separation probably caused tearing of the adjacent articular capsules with subsequent formation of the communication. The transverse channel allowing communication between L4–5 and L5–S1 bilaterally probably branched out from the medial side of the areas of spondylolysis, where diverticular dilatations were seen in three other patients. These dilatations might represent an extension of the inferior recess normally located in this area. Both increased pressure within these abnormal cavities and repeated tearing of their walls could explain their progressive enlargement. The inferior recess probably represents a weak area, as this is where leaking contrast material usually is seen after overdistention during arthrography. Periarticular leakage may be extensive, extending as far as the epidural space.[9]

Four of the 51 patients without spondylolysis reported transient radicular pain during distention of the facet joint which subsided immediately after reducing injection pressure or aspirating the contrast material. These four patients were later found to have a posterolateral disc herniation that displaced the nerve root toward the anteromedial aspect of the facet joint. Six of the 11 patients with spondylolysis had significant relief (75% to 100%) from their initial complaints; however, in all but two patients, pain recurred within 4 months. Those patients undergoing facet arthrography without spondylolysis showed that more than 50% had positive immediate results declining to less than 20% after 6 months.[9]

TECHNIQUE

Technically the performance of a successful facet injection is not difficult if the curved oblique orientation of the lower lumbar facet joints is taken into consideration during needle positioning. If viewed from above in the axial plane, the joints are angled laterally from anterior to posterior with a slight to marked anterolateral convexity. Viewed fluoroscopically from a lateral oblique orientation, the anterior and posterior bony margin of the facet joint can be identified with the patient in varying degrees of obliquity. This is important to realize, as many unsuccessful injections occur when the needle is directed toward the joint when it actually was embedded in the bone of the lateral aspect of the superior articular surface as it curves around the joint. This difficulty can be avoided by simply placing the patient prone during initial fluoroscopy and then gradually rotating the patient to one side. When the anterior and posterior walls of the facet joint can first be visualized, that represents the most posterior aspect of the joint where the needle can enter the joint. The easiest way to see the orientation of the facets with regard to angle of needle introduction is to look at facet joints on CT scans of the lumbar spine.

The use of local anesthetic is a matter of personal preference. Twenty-two gauge needles are used. Because of the duplicate innervation of the facet joints, the lower three facet joints are injected bilaterally if the pain does not localize, and unilaterally if it does. By adding a slight curve to the tip of the needle some directional control may be exerted. Occasionally the tip will enter the facet only after "walking" the needle around the area of the posterior joint space. Due to the curved shape of the facet joint, deep penetration into the joint often does not occur.

Once the needle is positioned, the facets are injected with steroids and a long-acting anesthetic agent such as Marcaine, 0.5%. Initially we used a mixture of 80 mg (40 mg/mL) of Depo-Medrol and 10 mL of 0.5% Marcaine, injecting 2 mL of this solution into each facet joint. During mixture of the two solutions, however, flocculation could be identified, and after deposits of whitish material could be identified in the facets at surgery, their use was stopped. (This finding is discussed in the article on epidural steroid injections.) An injection of 8 mg of Aristospan followed by 2 mL of 0.5% Marcaine or 0.5% Sensorcaine is used.

There is no flocculation of the Aristospan in the presence of the anesthetic agents.

With the exception of facet joints completely surrounded by osteophytes or postoperative changes, attempts are made to achieve intraarticular injections. One study specifically studied the efficacy of intraarticular versus extraarticular injections. The results showed that the injection of steroids was far more effective when done intraarticularly than extraarticularly. The authors felt that because there was a 56% rate of partial or complete relief at 6 months, the synovial lined lumbar facet joints are largely responsible for the facet syndrome.[8]

One purpose of the lumbar facet injection is to evaluate the change in the patient's clinical pain after the injection of anesthetic into the facet joint. In many patients, the relief of clinical back pain and occasionally radicular leg and hip pain shows a high degree of probability that their clinical pain is directly related to facet arthropathy, and this information can aid in determining the patient's prognosis and future course of action. No relief of pain indicates that the facet joints are probably not related to the patient's pain. If satisfactory, albeit temporary, relief occurs, an additional two injections for a total of three injections has been advocated.[6]

Morbidity of this procedure is minimal and is primarily confined to local tenderness at needle insertion sites, as indicated by other authors as well.[6] Failure to enter the facet joint is usually due to large osteophytes.

The mechanism by which the facet joint injection works is multifaceted. During contrast arthrography, there is frequent rupture of the inferior part of the capsule during or after injection. If leakage occurs on the lateral side, the contrast diffuses into the surrounding soft tissues where the branches of the posterior ramus of the spinal nerve pass. The importance of these branches in the innervation of the neural arch has been emphasized. If the leakage occurs on the medial side of the joint, through the ligamentum flavum, the drug spreads into the epidural space and sometimes into the intervertebral canal along the nerve root. As the steroids injected into the joint space follow the same course, the medication works not only on the synovial membrane, but eventually also on the adjacent nerve root. In addition, some of the effect of an epidural injection can be obtained.[2] Injection of the facet joints in patients with spondylolysis due to the intercommunication between the facet joints and the pars defect will result in effective dissemination of the medication into the pars defect as well as some epidural spread.[11]

CONCLUSION

Facet joint injections can be an effective treatment for the facet syndrome. Injections into the facet joint are probably more effective for long-term relief than are extraarticular injections.[8] Many patients with back pain, rather than disc herniation, may have pain due entirely or partially to facet arthropathy. Thus facet injections may serve a diagnostic as well as therapeutic role in the workup of back pain.

REFERENCES

1. Carrera GF: Lumbar facet arthrography and injection in low back pain. Wisconsin Med J 78:35–37, 1979.
2. Dory MA: Arthrography of the lumbar facet joints. Radiology 140:23–27, 1981.
3. Fairbank JCT, Park WM, McCall IW, O'Brien JP: Apophyseal injection of local anesthetic as a diagnostic aid in primary low-back pain syndromes. Spine 6:598–605, 1981.
4. Hickey RFJ, Tregonning, GD: Denervation of spinal facet joints for treatment of chronic low back pain. New Zealand Med J Feb:96–99, 1977.

5. Lau LSW, Littlejohn GO, Miller MH: Clinical evaluation of intra-articular injections for lumbar facet joint pain. Med J Austral 143:563–565, 1985.
6. Lewinnek GE, Warfield CA: Facet joint degeneration as a cause of low back pain. Clin Orthop 213:216–222, 1986.
7. Lippit AB: The facet joint and its role in spine pain. Spine 9:746–750, 1984.
8. Lynch MC, Taylor JF: Facet joint injection for low back pain. Bone Joint Surg 68B:138–141, 1986.
9. Maldaque B, Mathurin P, Malghem J: Facet joint arthrography in lumbar spondylolysis. Radiology 140:29–36, 1981.
10. McCall IW, Park WM, O'Brien JP: Induced pain referral from posterior lumbar elements in normal subjects. Spine 4:441–446, 1979.
11. Park WM, McCall IW, Benson D, et al: Spondyloarthrography: the demonstration of spondylolysis by apophyseal joint arthrography. Clin Radiol 36:427–430, 1985.

BARRY JEFFRIES, MD

EPIDURAL STEROID INJECTIONS

From the Department of Radiology, Georgia Baptist Hospital, Atlanta, Georgia

Reprint requests to:
Barry Jeffries, MD
Department of Radiology
Georgia Baptist Hospital
300 Boulevard, NE
Atlanta, GA 30312

The patient with acute or chronic back pain is a common therapeutic problem for the surgeon and diagnostic problem for the radiologist. The use of epidural steroid injections has gained widespread acceptance as a nonoperative treatment for back pain that can provide lasting relief of symptoms.

PATHOPHYSIOLOGY

Back pain with or without radicular pain can have one or several causes. The classic etiology of back pain with radicular symptoms is a herniated lumbar intervertebral disc directly compressing an adjacent nerve root. In response to the mechanical irritation, a local inflammatory response surrounding the disc and the nerve root contributes significantly to the radicular pain associated with disc herniation.[6] This local inflammatory response is felt to be secondary to degradation products from the degenerated herniated disc and is slow to resolve. If allowed to continue, it may cause intraneural and extraneural fibrosis, leading to chronic changes and symptoms.[12]

The role of inflammation and edema in back pain is demonstrated by the fact that inflamed nerve roots are sensitive to minor manipulation, whereas uninflamed nerve roots can be manipulated with minimal discomfort.[9] Improvement in clinical symptoms has been shown to coincide with reduction or resolution of nerve root edema without removal of the adjacent herniated disc.[2] Local irritation of nerve roots produces "H" substances at the site of injury, which are known to initiate pain. Cortisone is known to inhibit the peripheral response to "H" substances.[5] Brown[5] stated that epidural Depo-Medrol in patients with classic discogenic syndromes and symptoms of less than three months' duration had an excellent chance for symptomatic relief, supporting the theory that symptom production in the acute patient is mediated through an inflammatory mechanism. He felt the reason patients with chronic pain did not do well was because of the development of other causes for pain such as fibrosis. Many patients receiving epidural injections during the acute phase of their symptoms remained free of symptoms for long periods of time (up to 40 months), despite the fact that therapeutic levels of steroids are present within the epidural space for approximately 2 weeks. Brown concluded that pain in the acute disc syndrome was caused by the release of neural inflammatory substances caused by the chemical degeneration of the disc, and that long-lasting effects of the corticosteroids beyond the therapeutic life of the drug in the epidural space were due to the periodic rather than the continuous release of the inflammatory substances.

The inflammatory component of disc herniation or spinal stenosis with associated edema of the adjacent nerve roots justifies the use of corticosteroids in the treatment of back pain.[1,6,7,9] The corticosteroid agent reduces the amount of the inflammatory byproducts of disc herniation as well as the edema of the adjacent roots. As the root and the amount of adjacent soft tissues are reduced in size, there is less chance of recompression of the root as well as further production of degenerative byproducts. In patients with postoperative scarring, the corticosteroid agent may be effective due to its breakdown of collagen fibers.[4]

Degeneration or bulging of the disc usually results in narrowing of the disc space and subsequent osteophyte formation. The bulging disc and the osteophytes can compress the adjacent neural structures, with pain occurring in a manner similar to direct compression by a disc herniation.[1] Degenerative osteophytes and bony hypertrophy can also occur secondary to facet arthropathy or spondylolysis. These degenerative bony changes may directly cause back pain and radiculopathy from the degenerative changes or by compression of the nerve contained in the adjacent intervertebral canal. In spondylolysis, proliferative fibrocartilage may compress the nerve roots in the lateral recesses of the vertebral canal. With associated spondylolisthesis, the nerve roots may be stretched under the pedicle of the involved vertebral body and compressed between the superior posterior aspect of the disc and the inferior aspect of the pedicle.[1,13]

Patients who have had surgery for disc herniation or bony stenosis of the vertebra may develop symptoms after surgery that, in the absence of recurrent or residual disc herniation, are secondary to postoperative scarring. Patients who have had intradiscal chymopapain injection may develop mild narrowing of the disc or a sterile discitis. The reduction in disc height reduces the size of the adjacent intervertebral canals with subsequent edema of the nerve root secondary to compression.

TYPE OF INJECTION

Both epidural and intradural injections of steroids have been used for back pain and sciatica. The use of intradural steroid injection is controversial. Dullerud and Morland (1976) noted that 15 of 21 patients studied by myelography using Dimer-X plus Depo-Medrol developed arachnoiditis.[6a] Eighteen cases of arachnoiditis were reported by Roche in which the intrathecal injection of steroids was the only procedure or the procedure most likely to have been responsible for the arachnoiditis.[11] In Bernat's review of intradural corticosteroid injection, the treatment was used for lumbar radiculopathy, arachnoiditis, post-lumbar puncture, and multiple sclerosis. Complications included infections, aseptic meningitis, and adhesive arachnoiditis. The latter complications were related to intradural steroid injections for the treatment of neurologic conditions, particularly multiple sclerosis, and were felt to be dose related.[6] Many corticosteroids contain polyethylene glycol, a non-ionic detergent felt to cause aseptic meningitis and arachnoiditis. Bernat wrote that "Depo-Medrol is known clinically, pathologically and experimentally to cause meningeal inflammation after intrathecal injection."[11] Although intradural injection of corticosteroids has yet to be proven conclusively to be a major problem, this route of administration should probably be discontinued, particularly since there is evidence that it is less effective than epidural administration.[6]

Epidural administration of corticosteroids has been the most widely utilized method of administration. Either the translumbar or trans-sacral route may be employed.[6] Although the caudal approach can be effective if enough volume is injected, the lumbar approach allows the medication to be directly placed at the site of the suspected lesion.[1]

Lievre et al., in 1953, first used extradural injection of hydrocortisone for the relief of sciatica, followed by Goebert's report in the English literature 7 years later.[6] In one study, 80% of 30 patients treated with extradural corticosteroid-lignocaine mixture had excellent pain relief, whereas only 16% of 19 patients had excellent pain relief after injection of lignocaine alone.[4] In another study of 367 patients, good to excellent pain relief approaching 70% occurred in patients with subacute radicular leg pain (less than three months' duration) and chronic leg pain (more than three months duration) with no prior surgery. Negative myelograms and electromyograms in the absence of reflex or motor deficits also pointed toward optimal results. Patients with chronic pain who had prior surgery did less well. Patients for whom litigation was pending or who were receiving workmen's compensation generally had good to excellent results in 42–44% of cases as opposed to 64% of patients not undergoing litigation or receiving workmen's compensation. This finding suggests that a less optimal result may be expected in patients receiving compensation or undergoing litigation.[3]

In a review article by Benzon, several studies indicated that, although epidural steroid injection was effective in patients with chronic back pain, the response rate was better in those patients whose back pain was of short duration. Success rates ranged from 83–100% when the back pain was 3 months or less and 67–81% when the back pain was 6 months or less. Patients with back pain for less than 1 year had a success rate of 69% compared to 46% for those with pain duration over 1 year. Although the initial success rate was 85–90% for both chronic and acute back pain, at 6 months the success rate was 34% for acute pain and 12% for chronic pain. In general, patients responding to treatment (96%) did so within 6 days.[1] White et al. concluded that although 87% of selected patients had short-term relief and 34% had relief for as long as 6 months, there were no permanent cures in long-term follow-up.[16]

Epidural steroid injections are effective for back pain secondary to disc space narrowing, spondylolysis or spondylolisthesis, trauma, and after laminectomy. The common factor in these different causes of back pain appears to be irritation of the nerve root.[1] The success of epidural injection of corticosteroids in pain management is through relief of pressure on the nerve by shrinking reactive scar tissue and by direct reduction of nerve root edema. The role of epidural steroid injection in the presence of abnormal bone structure is less clear. The development of radiologic changes in the spine diminishes the possibility of improvement, as the steroids will not alter the bone structure compressing the nerves. In spite of the theoretical limitations above, in one study 60% of 75 patients with degenerative changes of the spine noted improvement compared to 63% of patients without changes on x-ray. Although the initial success rate from an epidural steroid injection in patients with disc and bone abnormalities was the same (81–90%), continued relief at 6 months was only 3.7–10% in the patients with disc syndrome compared to 0–1.5% in the patients with spinal stenosis, spondylolysis, and spondylolisthesis. The poor long-term results are probably due to the continuing mechanical pressure on the nerve roots by the bony abnormality that results in recurrent nerve inflammation and fibrosis.[1] We have begun epidural steroid injections into the cervical epidural space primarily for spondylosis. In spite of severe bony changes, two patients had a reduction of symptoms after the initial injections.

In patients after laminectomy, a success rate of 76% after three epidural steroid injections has been reported, but this high rate of success has not been equaled. Brown reported a 15% improvement in these patients. Patients with a new radiculopathy or involvement of nerve roots other than those involved initially responded best. The poor results are probably due to postoperative epidural scarring around the nerve roots, arachnoiditis, and the chronicity of pain.[1] Pheasant and Dyck stated that use of epidural steroid injections in the failed back syndrome patient were temporizing measures.[10]

Complications after epidural steroid injections have been minor. Headache, dizziness, transient hypotension, and worsening of the pain in the back or leg are related to the volume or speed of the injection. Rare, serious complications include septic or aseptic meningitis, worsening of symptoms of multiple sclerosis, and arachnoiditis. The most serious complications were related to intrathecal administration of the steroid.[1,14] Salt and water retention resulting in Cushing's syndrome have been reported. For this reason, a maximum dose not to exceed 3 mg/kg of Depo-Medrol has been recommended. Other complications include congestive heart failure due to salt and water retention, epidural abscess, and intraocular hemorrhage.[1] Intraocular hemorrhage occurred after rapid injection of 120 ml of saline. Large amounts of saline were previously recommended to be injected to break down fibrous adhesions between the dural sheaths of the nerve roots and the foramina, or to displace the nerve roots away from the disc. The large volumes injected caused headache and pain, probably mediated through compression of the subarachnoid space. A large volume is not necessary as 6 ml of radiopaque contrast spread from L1 to S5 in the epidural space.[1] It is also unlikely that a simple injection of fluid, most of which passes out of the intervertebral foramen, will break down dense scar tissue difficult to dissect during surgery.[15]

Dilution of the steroid serves another purpose. In rats, degenerative lesions in sciatic nerves occurred after exposure to polyethylene glycol contained in corticosteroid preparations. Dilution, therefore, reduces the concentration of the chemical and reduces the chance of morbidity. The steroid can be diluted with either saline or local anesthetic with no detectable change in the success rate. The addition of local anesthetic has been advocated to break the cycle of pain.[1] However, local anesthetic will cause some steroids such as Depo-Medrol to flocculate. No study of the consequences of the flocculation of the medication on either the efficacy of the treatment or the injected soft tissues has been done. As the effects are not known, it would seem reasonable that if Depo-Medrol is used, dilution with normal saline to a volume of 5–10 ml might be reasonable. Aristospan, a triamcinolone hexacetonide suspension does not contain polyethylene glycol, and dilution is not necessary.

Epidural steroid injection should not be performed in the presence of infection, bleeding diathesis or anticoagulation, known hypersensitivity to corticosteroids, the cauda equina syndrome, a progressive neural deficit, multiple sclerosis, or before a definitive diagnosis of acute disc prolapse is reached.[6,14] If two or three previous injections have failed to produce a prolonged benefit, additional injections are not warranted; there has been no additional relief after the initial three injections.[1] Indiscriminate use or use in patients whose symptoms are psychological is not advised.[6]

TECHNIQUE OF INJECTION

In our institution, the translumbar approach for placement of epidural steroids is utilized, as a smaller dose and volume can be employed to attain therapeutic levels at the site of suspected pathology. The patient's plain films, myelograms, CT scans, and MR studies of the back are evaluated. Because most epidural injections are done by radiologists, correlation of the level requested by the referring physician with the level indicated on the initial studies is mandatory. If any discrepancy is encountered, the referring physician is consulted before the injection.

The patient is placed prone on the fluoroscopic table and the back is fluoroscopically evaluated to identify the site of injection. Special care must be taken to correctly identify the level of pathology in patients with transitional vertebrae or postoperative changes. The skin is prepared and draped, and 1% Xylocaine is used as a local anesthetic. A midline puncture is always performed to take advantage of the increased resistance to injection of air by the interspinous ligaments, unless a fusion makes a posterolateral approach mandatory. Although special blunt needles and 18 gauge needles have been advocated for epidural placement of medication, we use 22 gauge spinal needles. Although there is theoretically a greater chance of puncturing the dura with the smaller diamond-tipped needle, the cutting edge of the spinal needle is sufficiently less sharp than a regular hypodermic needle that perforation of the dura occurs in only a small number of patients. Even so, with the small caliber of the needle, the probability of postprocedural headache is low, as the incidence of headache after spinal tap is lower with 22 gauge as opposed to 18 gauge needles.

The needle is advanced under fluoroscopic guidance with the central stylet in place until it is firmly within the interspinous ligament; this can be felt as a relatively greater resistance to the advancement of the needle compared to the subcutaneous tissues. At this point the stylet is removed and a 20 cc plastic syringe is attached to the needle. A well-lubricated glass syringe can also be used. A 20 cc syringe is used because a smaller volume syringe would allow greater pressure to be exerted through the needle for the same pressure applied to the plunger. With the larger syringe and the smaller gauge needle, the difference between the pressure required to inject air into the interspinous ligament or paraspinous muscles and the pressure required to inject air into the epidural space is relatively greater than the pressure difference using a smaller syringe and larger needle. Pressure is exerted on the plunger of the syringe and, if the needle is properly placed, upon release of the pressure the plunger will withdraw spontaneously, indicating no air injection. Pressure is then reapplied and the needle is carefully advanced. This work can be monitored fluoroscopically, but we usually do not in an effort to decrease the radiation dose.

Generally, resistance of the interspinous ligament indicates a continued midline course. When the potential epidural space is entered, there is a discernible decrease in the force necessary to inject air. The falling-drop method of determining entry into the epidural space is not felt to be sensitive enough due to the small size of the needle and its relatively high resistance to flow of fluids. Once entry into the epidural space is suspected, suction is applied to the syringe to exclude the possibility of inadvertent entry into the subarachnoid space. One of the advantages of the falling-resistance method of determining entry into the epidural space is that air injection pushes the dura away from the needle.

Should entry into the subarachnoid space occur, the needle can be withdrawn and a puncture done at an adjacent level. In patients where the pressure of air injection indicates probable entry into the epidural space, but the force of injection is greater than that normally encountered, a small injection of contrast material is indicated to confirm entry into the epidural space. The contrast material should flow from the needle in an irregular pattern. If it remains around the needle or assumes a linear shape, it is in the adjacent ligamentous or muscular structures. If it forms a homogeneous, poorly marginated collection, it is probably subarachnoid. Use of contrast material is essential for proper needle placement in those patients injected after surgery or with spinal stenosis, as the epidural space will probably be compressed or obliterated by scarring and a definite injection of air will be unlikely. If injection of contrast material is necessary, one of the non-ionic contrast solutions should be used because of their low potential for neurologic sequelae and no significant potential for causing arachnoiditis. One of the essential procedural requirements of the epidural steroid injection is the proper placement of the needle. In one study, 25% of the initial needle placements were incorrect; usually they were positioned posterior to the epidural space.[15]

If injections are to be made into the cervical epidural space, a slight modification of the above technique is necessary. The soft tissues and ligaments provide less resistance to the introduction of air into the posterior epidural space, and initial attempts to determine entry into the epidural space using the falling-resistance method were unsuccessful, as the needle was positioned too far posteriorly. As a result, after initial introduction of the needle approximately 2 cm into the midline posterior soft tissues of the neck, the patient is turned to a left lateral decubitus position and the needle advanced until its tip is slightly anterior to the posterior aspect of the vertebral canal, as determined by the posterior laminar line. At this point the patient is turned prone, needle aspiration done to exclude entry into the subarachnoid space, and there is an injection of Omnipaque 180. If typical spread of the contrast within the epidural space occurs, then the steroid is introduced. If not, the needle is alternately advanced, aspirated, and injected until the epidural space is entered as determined by injection of contrast. Due to the size and proximity of the cervical spinal cord, greater care is necessary to avoid inadvertent puncture of the subarachnoid space or direct injury to the cord itself.

INJECTABLE AGENTS

Once proper placement of the needle is confirmed, the corticosteroid is injected. Many variations in the amount and type of injections have been used: 80 mg Depo-Medrol diluted in 5 ml of lidocaine;[6] 80 mg Depo-Medrol;[6] 80 mg Depo-Medrol in 10 ml normal saline;[6] adcortyl 10 mg in 1 ml Xylocaine;[4] 40 mg Depo-Medrol in 1 ml lignocaine;[4] 100 mg Depo-Medrol in 10 ml of 0.5% Sensorcaine;[3] 100 mg hydrocortisone in 10 ml of 0.5% Sensorcaine;[3] 120 mg Depo-Medrol in 3 ml of 1% Xylocaine;[5] 120 Depo-Medrol in 10 ml of 0.25% Marcaine;[16] and 4–6 ml of normal saline followed by 80 mg of Depo-Medrol.[8]

As indicated by the wide diversity in amount and types of mixtures, there is no single best technique. We initially injected either 1 ml of 80 mg/ml or 2 ml of 40 mg/ml Depo-Medrol mixed with 5 ml of 0.5% Marcaine. Mixture of these agents results in flocculation that can be seen in the syringe. One surgeon who used the epidural steroid injection noted that at surgery in patients who had received previous injections there were collections of white material at the injection site. These collections probably represent unabsorbed medication, although some of the material may represent a host response. In addition, one of the physicians inadvertently injected the steroid-Marcaine mixture into the subarachnoid space, which resulted in paralysis of the lower extremities for approximately 5 hours. For these reasons, the mixture of Depo-Medrol and a local anesthetic is no longer used.

We have been using the corticosteroid Aristospan. Our injections are 1 ml of 20 mg/ml. Although local anesthetics can be mixed with this steroid without flocculation, we prefer to keep the dose as concentrated as possible at the site of pathology and to avoid the risk of inadvertent subarachnoid injection. Because there is no ethylene glycol in the administered dose, there is no potential risk to the adjacent neural structures during use of undiluted medication.

Most of our patients treated in this manner are outpatients. Complications include headache after spinal tap due to inadvertent entry into the subarachnoid space (6 cases), transient radicular discomfort in the legs due to pressure exerted on the thecal sac by the epidural mass effect of the steroid (1 case), and temporary paralysis of the lower extremities caused by inadvertent injection of the steroid-Marcaine solution into the thecal sac (1 case). Because we average 10 cases per week, this is a low rate of morbidity.

In our institution, epidural steroid injections have been requested for patients with acute disc herniations, congenital spinal stenosis associated with achondroplasia, epidural scarring secondary to laminectomy, spondylosis (both lumbar and cervical), and radicular pain after chymopapain therapy for herniated disc. Although we have not formally studied the efficacy of epidural steroid treatment, our results, based on discussions with our referring surgeons, would indicate initial results comparable with the above studies. There has also been some long-term relief, particularly in patients with acute symptoms such as the radiculopathy after chymopapain injection. Because this is felt to be related to a chemical discitis, the acute negation of the effects of disc breakdown byproducts by the epidural steroid is the probable cause. There was also initial success after epidural steroid injection into a tightly stenotic vertebral canal of an achondroplastic dwarf. The long-term results of the treatment have yet to be determined.

CONCLUSION

The injection of corticosteroids into the epidural space for the treatment of back pain can be useful in many applications. The technique appears to work best for acute lesions related to nerve root edema secondary to disc pathology. It can occasionally relieve symptoms in patients with chronic back problems, but the long-term prognosis is less favorable. The procedure is safe and can be easily done on an outpatient basis.

REFERENCES

1. Benzon HT: Epidural steroid injections for low back pain and lumbosacral radiculopathy. Pain 24:277–295, 1986.

2. Berg A: Clinical and myelographic studies of conservatively treated cases of lumbar intervertebral disc protrusion. Acta Chir Scand 104:124–129, 1953.

3. Berman AT, Garbarino JL Jr, Fisher SM, Bosacco SJ: The effects of epidural injection of local anesthetics and corticosteroids on patients with lumbosciatic pain. Clin Orthop 188:144–151, 1984.

4. Bourne IHJ: Treatment of chronic back pain. Practitioner 228:333–338, 1984.

5. Brown FW: Management of diskogenic pain using epidural and intrathecal steroids. Clin Orthop 129:72–78, 1977.

6. Corrigan AB, Carr G, Tugwell S: Intraspinal corticosteroid injections. Med J Austral Mar:224–225, 1982.

7. Green LN: Dexamethasone in the management of symptoms due to herniated lumbar disc. J Neurol Neurosurg Psychiat 38:1211–1217, 1975.

8. Green PWB, Addison JB, Weiss CA, Langan P: The role of epidural cortisone injection in the treatment of diskogenic low back pain. Clin Orthop 153:121–125, 1980.

9. Murphy RW: Nerve roots and spinal nerves in degenerative disk disease. Clin Orthop 129:46–60, 1977.

10. Pheasant HC, Dyck P: Failed lumbar disc surgery. Clin Orthop 164:93–108, 1982.

11. Roche J: Steroid-induced arachnoiditis. Med J Austral Mar:281–284, 1984.

12. Ryan MD, Taylor TKF: Management of lumbar nerve-root pain by intrathecal and epidural injections of depot methylprednisolone acetate. Med J Austral Nov:532–533, 1951.

13. Seimon LP: Low Back Pain: Clinical Diagnosis and Management. Norwalk, CT, Appleton-Century-Crofts, 1983, pp 3–114.

14. Stambough JL, Booth RE, Rothman RH: Transient hypercorticism after epidural steroid injection. Bone Joint Surg 66A:1115–1116, 1984.

15. White AH: Injection techniques for the diagnosis and treatment of low back pain. Orthoped Clin North Am 14:553–567, 1983.

16. White AH, Derby R, Wynne G: Epidural injections for the diagnosis and treatment of low-back pain. Spine 5:78–86, 1980.

RICHARD W. FOSTER, MD

COMPUTED TOMOGRAPHY OF SPINAL TRAUMA

From the Section of Neuroradiology, Department of Radiology, Tulane University Medical Center, New Orleans, Louisiana

Reprint requests to:
Richard W. Foster
Department of Radiology
Tulane University Medical Center
1430 Tulane Avenue
New Orleans, LA 70112

The use of computed tomography (CT) in the evaluation of spinal trauma has received considerable attention in the literature. The advent of CT has opened important new dimensions in the evaluation of the spine in trauma, and some authors have stated the greatest use of spinal CT is in the trauma setting.

CT is considered the method of choice in the evaluation of spinal trauma. Its advantages over plain film examination are well documented. Plain films can often underestimate bone and soft tissue injury, and not all fractures of the spine are clearly delineated by routine radiographs. CT can provide information not available on plain radiographs and can detect fractures and displaced fragments that may be missed. CT is superior to plain films for bony detail and can assess associated soft tissue damage with greater accuracy.

INDICATIONS AND TECHNIQUE

CT examination should not be utilized as a screening tool for spinal injury; it is indicated in those patients who present with neurological deficits and in those whose plain radiographs are suggestive of or demonstrate spinal abnormality. Preliminary AP and lateral plain films are recommended prior to CT examination for adequate evaluation of the extent of trauma. The study should be tailored to include adjacent levels of normal to insure examination completeness. Computer generated radiographs (scout views, pilot views, scanograms, etc.) in the sagittal plane allow proper gantry angulation, which should be perpendicular to the spinal canal.

In the cervical region, continuous 1.5 mm thick sections are recommended for thorough examination. Very thin sections will lessen the chance of subtle abnormalities being overlooked due to volume averaging. In addition, thinner sectioning will increase the resolution of reformatted images in other planes. For the remainder of the spine, 4 or 5 mm thick sections at 3 mm table increments are recommended. The overlapping sections will also lend to higher resolution in reformatted images.

Coronal and sagittal reconstructions should be obtained routinely in the evaluation of spinal trauma. This is a must. Abnormalities of alignment (often quite subtle), which may be overlooked in axial images, can be detected and defined with the aid of reformatted images (Fig. 1). The importance of these "free" images cannot be overstated. They are mandatory in the evaluation of spinal trauma.

High-resolution bone reconstruction algorithms should be employed in the CT examination of spinal trauma. These programs produce images of exquisite bony detail, which decreases the chances of missing subtle abnormalities. Imaging should be performed at narrow- and wide-window settings for proper examination of both the soft tissues and osseous structures.

Motion control is extremely important even with state-of-the-art scanners and very fast scan times. If the patient moves between scans, a fracture may be entirely missed. Motion during exposures will render the axial slices uninterpretable and decrease the reliability of sagittal and coronal reformatted images. Sedation or general anesthesia has been recommended; however, in patients with associated head injuries, this may be inadvisable.

Finally, from the technical standpoint, CT scans of patients with acute spinal trauma should be performed with the radiologist in attendance. It is his or her responsibility to prescribe the scan, monitor the images, and obtain appropriate additional slices, thinner slices, reformatted images, etc. Imaging of the acute traumatic spine is not a routine scan for simple low back pain with radiculopathy where the radiologist's presence is not critical. The study needs to be carefully planned, executed, and interpreted in a timely and orderly fashion to insure proper patient management.

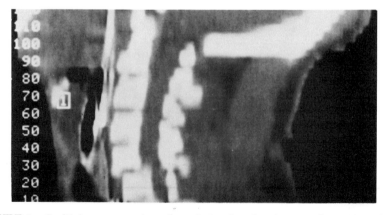

FIGURE 1. Sagittal reconstruction of cervical spine showing anterior subluxation of C5 on C6. This was not as apparent on axial images.

ADVANTAGES

The advantages of CT in the evaluation of spinal trauma are legion and have been well documented. CT is a quick, safe, easy, comfortable, noninvasive way to evaluate the spine without subjecting the patient to additional movement that may cause further damage. This is especially important in patients with severe spinal injuries and in those who present with neurologic deficits. Plain film evaluation, including tomography, often requires patient manipulation, which can be deleterious; CT obviates this additional movement.

The ability of CT to assess the spine in the axial plane is ideal. Not only can the vertebral bodies be examined, but the integrity of the spinal canal and neural foramina may also be addressed. CT can evaluate the size and configuration of the neural canal and detect compromise due to the presence of subluxation/dislocation, retropulsed fragments, or other foreign bodies such as bullet fragments. Axial imaging is also ideal for evaluation of the osseous posterior elements. Fractures of the pedicles, lamina, and spinous processes are readily apparent. The integrity of the facet joints may also be evaluated; subtle abnormalities such as distracted facets should alert one to the presence of unstable fracture, dislocation or ligamentous injury. Ununited facets or dislocated facets should be easily recognized.

Examination of the paraspinal soft tissues may also be performed with CT, another great advantage of this modality over plain film radiography. The presence of transverse process fracture in a patient with upper lumbar spinal trauma should alert one to the possibility of renal damage, and close scrutiny of the kidneys should be undertaken. Likewise, thoracolumbar trauma with associated rib fractures should lead to inspection of the liver and spleen to rule out laceration, subcapsular hematoma, etc. The location and extent of paravertebral hematomas associated with fractures may also be defined.

The intraspinal soft tissues may also be inspected with transaxial CT scanning. With the high resolution scanners available today, spinal cord hemorrhage/hematoma may be detected as a high-density focus within the cord. Epidural hematomas may also be seen as high-density collections adjacent to the cord. It is very important to differentiate these entities. Hematomyelia is treated conservatively, whereas an epidural hemorrhage usually requires more aggressive treatment. Epidural hematomas can severely compress the cord or cauda equina with rapid progression of symptoms. Surgical decompression is necessary or permanent neurologic deficits can occur. Cord edema is best seen on CT following intrathecal injection of a small amount of water soluble myelographic contrast. This can be fairly easily performed via a lateral C1–2 puncture.

Probably the greatest advantage of CT in the evaluation of spinal trauma is its ability to provide multiplanar reconstruction/reformatted images. This feature enables delineation of alignment abnormalities and classification of fracture dislocations. Neural canal compromise can be clearly defined in the axial plane as well as in the sagittal and/or coronal planes (Fig. 2). Horizontally oriented fractures involving the odontoid, vertebral bodies, or articular facets, which may be overlooked on axial images, are more likely to be detected utilizing reformatted images. Reformatted images aid in the identification of traumatic neural foraminal narrowing as well as locked or perched facets. Reconstruction images are vital components to the proper CT evaluation of spinal trauma; they should be obtained routinely. They are quickly performed at no additional radiation exposure to the patient.

Finally, CT delivers less radiation dosage to the patient than an equivalent

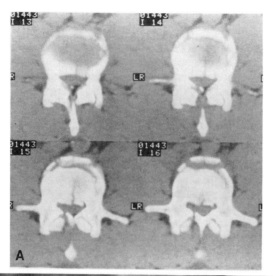

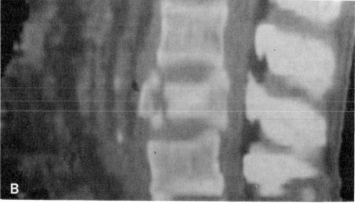

FIGURE 2.   Axial (*A*) and sagittal (*B*) reformatted images of an L3 compression fracture showing compromise of the neural canal by posteriorly displaced vertebral body fragments.

plain film tomographic examination. The information provided is similar to that of tomography; however, the ability to vary the gray scale makes CT easier to interpret and somewhat more sensitive. As stated previously, CT is certainly more comfortable and less potentially hazardous to the patient.

DISADVANTAGES

The limitations of CT in the evaluation of spinal trauma are few; however, some do exist. Probably the most important is the inability of axial CT to detect horizontally oriented fractures. This limitation has been documented in the odontoid region as well as in the articular pillars of the cervical spine. Subtle horizontal fractures of the vertebral bodies, pedicles, or laminae throughout the spine may also be overlooked. Likewise, minimal vertebral body compression fractures may not be detected on axial CT scans. Coronal and/or sagittal reformation images play an important role in minimizing these limitations.

Increases or decreases in disc space height are poorly appreciated on axial images. Subluxations and dislocations are also less obvious with transaxial scans. Longitudinal reformatted images are mandatory so these abnormalities are not missed.

Reformatted images have decreased contrast and spatial resolution compared to the original axial images. Even with the utilization of thin sections and overlapping sections, there is some loss of image quality.

The partial volume averaging effect may simulate fracture in some instances. This problem is lessened when thinner sectioning is used. Again longitudinal reformations can aid in minimizing this limitation.

POSTMYELOGRAPHY CT

Postmyelography CT (CTM) has proven to be a useful adjunct in the radiographic evaluation of radiculopathy, neck pain, low back pain, the failed back syndrome, and spinal infectious or metastatic disease. It can also be an important tool in the evaluation of spinal trauma. Complete myelographic examination need not precede CTM. A few milliliters of water–soluble contrast (Iohexol or Iopamidol with an iodine concentration of 180–240 mg/ml) can fairly easily be injected into the subarachnoid space either in the cervical or lumbar region depending on the site of injury. This should provide adequate opacification of the subarachnoid space for CT examination.

Traumatic lesions that can be more fully evaluated with CTM are numerous. Cord swelling secondary to edema or hemorrhage is better appreciated as thinning of the surrounding opacified subarachnoid space. Epidural hemorrhage/ hematoma or associated traumatic disc herniation may be displayed as displacement of the cord/cauda associated with attenuation of the subarachnoid space (Fig. 3). Total block may exist. Significant narrowing of the spinal canal with compression of the cord/cauda secondary to osseous encroachment from displaced fragments and subluxations is better visualized with this method (Figs. 4 and 5). Finally, dural tears and nerve root avulsions are more likely to be diagnosed with the use of CTM (Fig. 6).

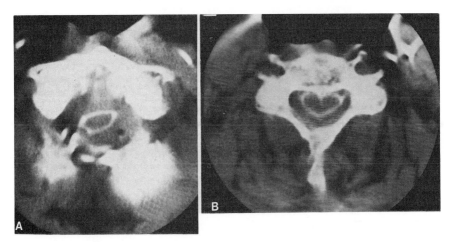

FIGURE 3. CTM of an extensive postoperative epidural hematoma with thecal sac attenuation at the region of the atlas (*A*) and more inferiorly at C3 (*B*).

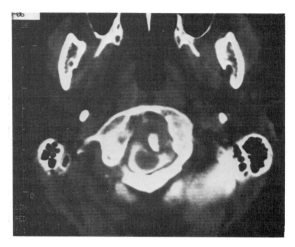

FIGURE 4. CTM showing marked anterior subluxation of the atlas with resulting compression of the cord in a patient with rheumatoid arthritis.

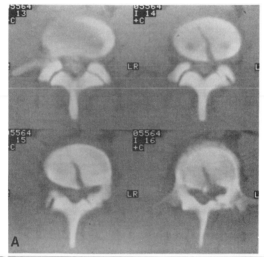

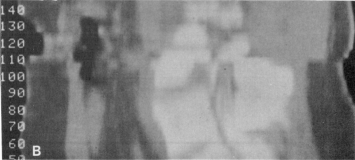

FIGURE 5. CTM of a compression fracture of L4. Multidisplay axial images (*A*) and sagittal reformatted image (*B*) showing attenuation and almost total block of the opacified thecal sac by retropulsed fragments.

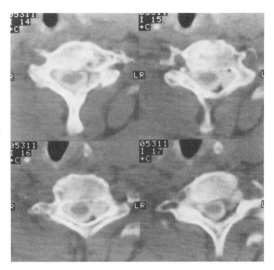

FIGURE 6. CTM showing fracture deformity at the C6 level with an extrathecal collection of contrast.

THREE DIMENSIONAL RECONSTRUCTION

A discussion of CT in spinal trauma would not be complete without some mention of 3-D reconstruction images. Most major manufacturers of CT and MRI have 3-D programs available or in development.

The process requires special software packages. Thin (1.5–3.0 mm), unangled axial images are necessary to produce reconstructions of fine detail. Axial data is converted and displayed to appear three dimensional by utilizing tinting or shadowing. The resulting 3-D images may then be rotated about any axis or transected along any axis to provide unique "fantastic-voyage-like" views of the areas of interest. It is obvious that patient cooperation is of the utmost importance. The patient must remain motionless during the scan. As with multiplanar reformation images, motion will distort 3-D reconstruction images with resultant loss of information.

This technique does not provide any new information but rather presents available data in a unique way. This method of display appears to be better understood by referring physician. It has already been utilized in clinical practice for the evaluation of spinal trauma, spinal infection, and the postoperative spine. Three-D reconstructions appear to be most useful in the evaluation and preoperative planning of complex bony injuries. They are of little use in the evaluation of associated soft tissue injuries.

MECHANISMS OF INJURY

Classic mechanisms have been enumerated to define traumatic injuries of the spinal column. These include flexion, extension, axial loading (vertical compression), rotation, distraction, and shearing. It must be emphasized that many traumatic injuries of the spine result from combinations of these mechanisms. A classic example is unilateral locked or perched facet resulting from hyperflexion in combination with rotation.

When dealing with spinal injuries, it should be remembered that one need not have radiographic evidence of osseous disruption of the spinal column in order to have significant neurologic injury. With hyperflexion, there may be significant instantaneous cord or cauda compression only to have the bony spine return to a normal configuration following the transient flexion forces. This is especially true in patients with degenerative or congenital canal stenosis where momentary flexion/extension can cause considerable cord/cauda compromise only to have subsequent normal-appearing radiographs. Knowledge of the mechanism of injury may lead to further evaluation such as CTM, where cord enlargement secondary to edema or hemorrhage is better appreciated. In addition, neurologic deficit without osseous disruption should make one highly suspicious of significant ligamentous injury.

Neurologic deficits are not only related to injury mechanisms but also to the velocities of the forces involved. Low velocity injuries such as low-speed automobile accidents, sporting injuries, and falls are usually associated with minor to moderate degrees of neurologic impairment. On the other hand, high-velocity injuries, such as high-speed motor vehicle accidents and gunshot injuries, are more commonly associated with more serious degrees of neurologic compromise.

ANATOMICAL CONSIDERATIONS

Traumatic injuries to the spinal column have been reported throughout its length from the cervicocranial junction to the coccyx. The majority of injuries occur in the regions of the highest mobility, specifically the lower cervical spine and the thoracolumbar junction. There are key anatomic reasons for the propensity of the injuries in these areas.

In the cervical spine, the articular facets are coronally oriented at approximately 45 degrees from the horizontal (Fig. 7A). This allows for a great deal of sliding motion with flexion and extension. At the thoracolumbar junction, the vertically and basically coronally oriented facets assume a more sagittal orientation, which also allows for greater motion with flexion and extension (Fig. 7B). The posterior ligaments (flava, capsular, interspinous, and supraspinous) are the limiting structures with forced hyperflexion or hyperextension.

The thoracic spine is somewhat stabilized due to its facet orientation and the surrounding rib cage. The facets are vertically and coronally oriented, allowing for very little motion in flexion and extension (Fig. 7C). Additionally, the strong costovertebral and costosternal attachments reinforce the spinal column and limit motion. Indeed, traumatic forces must be great to cause fractures or dislocations in the thoracic spine.

The lower lumbar spine is stabilized by the attachments of the psoas major muscles. In addition, the posterior ligaments are stronger and the intertransverse ligaments (between transverse processes) are more definable in this region than in the remainder of the spine. This combination tends to limit motion in the lower lumbar spine.

The sacrococcygeal spine is immobile and naturally braced by the bony pelvis. As in the thoracic spine, severe trauma is necessary to cause injury, which is usually associated with marked bony and soft tissue pelvic injury.

It is very important to understand facet relationships when interpreting spinal CT. They are normally very tightly apposed and quite symmetric in appearance. Facets should always be paired (superior and inferior). Any separation, asymmetry, or abnormal relationship should be viewed as highly suspicious evidence of significant spinal trauma (Fig. 8A). Thorough examination to exclude associated fractures and subluxations must be undertaken. Additionally, the uncovertebral joints in the cervical spine may show subtle asymmetry

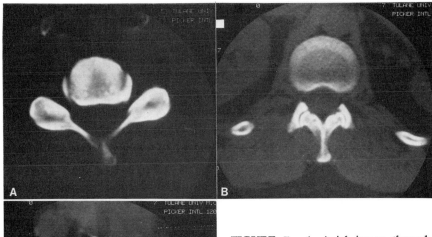

FIGURE 7. A, Axial image through midcervical region showing coronal orientation of the facet joints. Also note normal-appearing uncovertebral joints. *B,* Axial scan at the thoracolumbar junction demonstrating the sagittally oriented facets, which allows motion with flexion and extension. *C,* Axial slice at the level of the aortic arch showing coronally oriented facets. These facets are also vertically oriented (as opposed to the cervical region), which allows little motion.

which should raise a red flag (Fig. 8B). The importance of close inspection of these areas when dealing with spinal trauma cannot be overstated.

LONG-TERM FOLLOW-UP AND POSTOPERATIVE EXAMINATION

In dealing with the long-term follow-up of traumatic spinal injuries, several key points need to be addressed. These include patency of the spinal canal and neural foramina, development of syrinxes, and integrity or stability of fusions.

Significant canal or foraminal narrowing may occur secondary to posttraumatic osteophyte formation. Additionally, there may be stenosis as a result of bony fusions, wire fixations, or rod placements. CT is an excellent tool for the evaluation of such conditions. Narrowings caused by bony osteophytes or fusion fragments are easily identified. Even though wire suture material and fixation rods produce undesirable metallic streak artifacts, significant information can be gained utilizing a combination of thin axial scans and longitudinal reformations.

The integrity of bone grafts is best evaluated using coronal and sagittal reformation images. Pseudoarthroses or nonfusions should be readily identifiable when wide window settings are employed.

Probably the most important aspect in the long-term follow-up of a spinal injury patient is the demonstration of syrinx development. Typically, this occurs

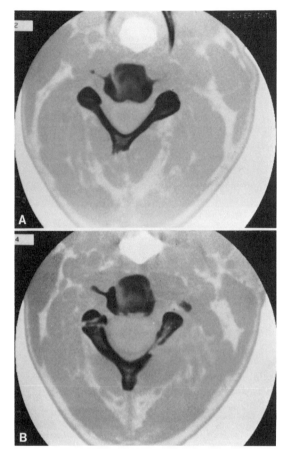

FIGURE 8. A, Section through midcervical region showing normally positioned facet joints. B, A section more cephalad demonstrating fracture dislocation of the right inferior facet associated with widening of the facet and uncovertebral joints.

some 4 to 5 years following injury and is heralded by the onset and progression of new neurologic deficits following a period of clinical quiescence. It is most important to make the diagnosis, because surgical intervention and shunting may stop symptom progression and in some cases have reversed or improved the neurologic deficits. The previous gold standard for the diagnosis of syrinx was delayed CTM. The collection of water-soluble contrast within the spinal cord is diagnostic for syringomyelia and myelomalacia (micro-cyst formation). MRI is now the preferred method for the evaluation of suspected syrinx formation as it is noninvasive and more sensitive.

CONCLUSION

CT is an ideal method for the evaluation of spinal trauma. CT is the procedure of choice; however, it should not be used as a screening examination. Patients who present with neurologic deficits or plain radiographic evidence of traumatic spinal abnormalities should be thoroughly evaluated with CT. It is safe, quick, and requires little additional movement that could prove detrimental to the patient. The ability of CT to provide multiplanar reformations as well as 3-D reconstructions enhances its diagnostic capabilities. CT is an excellent tool for the long-term follow-up of spinal trauma and the postoperative spine. The literature is replete with excellent articles dealing with CT in spinal trauma, and it is suggested that the reader examine the referenced articles for further study.

ACKNOWLEDGMENTS

The author would like to thank Mrs. Terry McGuckin and Mr. J. Richard Hutton for their assistance in the preparation of this manuscript.

REFERENCES

1. Atlas, SW, Regenbogen V, Rogers LF, et al: The radiographic characterization of burst fractures of the spine. AJNR 7:675–682, 1986.
2. Brant-Zawadski M, Jeffrey RB, Minagi H, et al: High resolution CT of thoracolumbar fractures. AJR 138:699–704, 1982.
3. Brant-Zawadski M, Miller EM, Federle MP: CT in the evaluation of spine trauma. AJR 136:369–375, 1981.
4. Cocayorin ED, Keiffer SA: Applications and limitations of computed tomography of the spine. Radiol Clin North Am 20:185–206, 1982.
5. Donovan-Post MJ, Green BA: The use of computed tomography in spinal trauma. Radiol Clin North Am 21:327–375, 1983.
6. Freiherr G: 3-D imaging in medicine: Synthesizing the third dimension. Diagn Imag 9:190–203, 1987.
7. Guerra J, Garfin SR, Resnick D: Vertebral burst fractures: CT analysis of the retropulsed fragment. Radiology 153:769–772, 1984.
8. Handel SF, Lee Y: Computed tomography of spinal fractures. Radiol Clin North Am 19:69–89, 1981.
9. Kilcoyne RF, Mack LA: Computed tomography of spinal fractures. Appl Radiol 16:40–54, 1987.
10. Manaster BJ, Osborn AG: CT patterns of facet fracture dislocations in the thoracolumbar region. AJNR 7:1007–1012, 1986.
11. Pech P, Kilgore DP, Pojunas KW, et al: Cervical spinal fractures: CT detection. Radiology 157:117–120, 1985.
12. Shuman WP, Rogers JV, Sickler ME, et al: Thoracolumbar burst fractures: CT dimensions of the spinal canal relative to postsurgical improvement. AJNR 6:337–341, 1985.
13. Woodring JH, Goldstein SJ: Fractures of the articular processes of the cervical spine. AJR 139:341–344, 1982.
14. Yetkin Z, Osborn AG, Giles DS, et al: Uncovertebral and facet joint dislocations in cervical articular pillar fractures: CT evaluation. AJNR 6:633–637, 1985.

AY-MING WANG, MD[1]
DAVID P. WESOLOWSKI, MD[2]
JALIL FARAH, MD[2]

EVALUATION OF POSTERIOR SPINAL STRUCTURES BY COMPUTED TOMOGRAPHY

[1]Department of Radiology, Brigham and Women's Hospital, Harvard Medical School, Boston, Massachusetts

[2]William Beaumont Hospital, Royal Oak, Michigan

Reprint requests to:
Ay-Ming Wang, MD
Department of Radiology
Brigham and Women's Hospital
75 Francis Street
Boston, MA 02115

The posterior spinal structures include as the bony portions of the pedicles, articular facets, laminae, and spinous process; and the ligamentous structures of the supraspinous and interspinous ligaments, ligamentum flava and strong capsular ligaments of the apophyseal joints. Stability of the spine depends on the integrity of these structures.[26] In the lumbar spine, the posterior elements are the key elements in the development of low-back pain or referred sciatica.[2,31,35,45]

High-resolution computed tomography (CT) allows excellent noninvasive evaluation of the bone and the adjacent soft tissues of the spine because of its high sensitivity and specificity for spinal pathology and excellent cross-section morphology. The pathology of the posterior spinal structures, including degenerative changes, spinal stenosis, trauma, primary bone neoplasm, metastatic disease, inflammatory process, spondylolysis, spondylolisthesis, and congenital anomalies, can be accurately studied by CT.[2,4–9,13–17,19–20,22,24–26,28–30,34,36–38,40–41,44–49,51] CT guidance of percutaneous biopsy can be done precisely and safely on an outpatient basis.[23] Sagittal, coronal, oblique plane, or detailed multiplanar reformatted images may facilitate the assessment of complicated bony anatomy.[16,44] Three-dimensional CT imaging provides significantly more information and better perception of bone abnormalities than 2-D CT imaging in spinal trauma,[14] but it is less useful in the study of the soft tissue alteration including thickening of ligamenta flava. High-resolution surface-coil magnetic resonance imaging (MRI) of the spine may have a complementary role in defining certain abnormalities such as congenital disorders, canal stenosis, and facet joint disorders in a noninvasive setting without the use of intrathecal contrast medium.[1,3,18,33–34,45]

TECHNICAL CONSIDERATIONS AND NORMAL CT ANATOMY

In the evaluation of a disorder of posterior spinal structures, a localization image (lateral and sometimes anteroposterior scout views) should always be obtained (Fig. 1). Patients are routinely placed supine on the scanner table. Scanning employs non-angled gantry, contiguous 4–5 mm thick sections at a 4–5 mm interval from the pedicle of the vertebra above and through the pedicle of the vertebra below the disc for evaluation of all osseous and soft tissue anatomy of the posterior spinal structures; additional contiguous 1.5–2 mm thick sections of angled gantry scanning parallel to the intervertebral disc at the disc levels is used selectively for evaluation of disc disease. Reformatted images may facilitate interpretation when applied to the assessment of the complicated bone anatomy. Multiple window and level settings should be used.

The spinal facet joints are a diarthrodial joint formed by the articulation of the concave surface of the anterolaterally located superior articular processes and the convex surface of the posteromedially located inferior articular processes. The joint has a very thin fibroelastic capsule attached at the osteocartilage junction; anteromedially the capsule is thickened by the lateral attachment of the ligamentum flavum. The capsule has superior and inferior recesses containing fat pads partially covered by a synovial tissue. Hyaline cartilage covers each facet and usually measures 2–4 mm in thickness. The ligamentum flavum extends

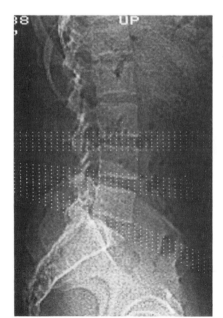

FIG 1. Lateral scout view of the lumbar spine reveals a protocol in which 2-mm thick sections to be obtained at 2-mm intervals through the neural foramina and intervertebral disc with the gantry angled selectively for true axial cuts.

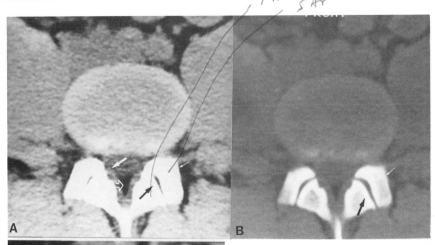

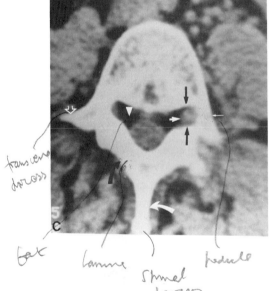

FIG 2. Normal lumbar axial CT scans. *A* and *B,* at L4-L5 disc, soft tissue setting and bone setting show the superior articular process of L5 (white arrow) anterolateral to the inferior articular process (black arrow). The facet capsule and anterior portion of the ligamentum flavum (large white arrow) cannot be separated. Epidural fat (open white arrow) lies between the ligamentum flavum. *C,* At L4, soft tissue setting shows L4 nerve root (white arrows) in the lateral recess (black arrows). The pedicle (thin white arrow), transverse process (open white arrow), epidural fat (white arrow head), lamina (curved black arrow) and spinal process (curved white arrow) are well identified.

from the anteroinferior border of the lamina above to the upper posterior border of the lamina below and measures 5 mm in thickness.

The posterior spinal structures can be accurately studied on CT scanning (Fig. 2) and may also be reliably studied on axial and sagittal MR images (Fig. 3).

SPINAL STENOSIS AND DEGENERATIVE DISEASE

Spinal Stenosis

Spinal stenosis is defined as a condition in which the size of the spinal canal or its lateral recess is reduced, causing compression of the dural sac and its contents. It occurs commonly in the lumbar and cervical regions and less commonly in the thoracic region. In the cervical and thoracic regions, stenosis causes spinal cord compression with or without nerve root compression. In the lumbar

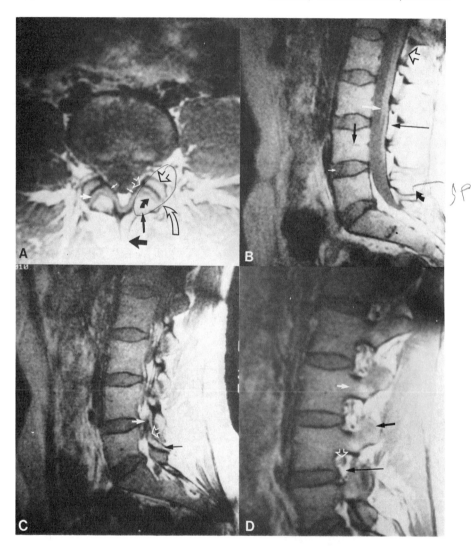

FIG 3. Normal MR imaging of lumbar spine. *A,* Axial T1-weighted MR image (SE 800/20) at L4-L5 level through both lamina (black arrow) and ligamenta flava (white arrows) separated by low-signal intensity of cortical bone. The superior articular facet (black open arrow), the inferior articular facet (curved black arrow) and the hyaline cartilage (large white arrow) between their cortical edges, lateral facet joint capsule (curved black open arrow), medial facet joint capsule (white open arrow) and spinal process (thick black arrow) are well identified. *B,* Midline T1-weighted sagittal MR image (SE 800/20) shows spinal process (curved black arrow), epidural fat (long black arrow), ligamentum flavum (black open arrow), cauda equina (white arrow), L4-L5 intervertebral disc (white arrow), and basivertebral vein channel (black arrow). *C,* Parasagittal T1-weighted MR image (SE 800/20) across medial facet plane shows superior articular facet (small white arrow), inferior articular facet (black arrow), and isthmus (white open arrow). *D,* Parasagittal T1-weighted MR image (SE 800/20) across pedicle plane shows pedicle (white arrow), dorsal root ganglia (white open arrow), epidural fat (long black arrow), and superior articular facet (black arrow).

region, it may cause low back pain, sciatica, and claudication pain with hyperextension of the back but not with flexion.

Spinal stenosis may be congenital (developmental) or acquired. The congenital type may be complicated by superimposed acquired disease.[11,12] Many patients with congenital spinal stenosis do not develop clinical symptoms and signs until acquired processes supervene. Congenital spinal stenosis includes the idiopathic variety, achondroplasia, and Morquio's syndrome. Spinal stenosis may be seen in patients with diastrophic dwarfism usually without clinical symptoms[5] (Fig. 4) and Klippel-Feil syndrome[40] (Fig. 5). Acquired spinal stenosis may be caused by degenerative disease (Fig. 6), some fractures and dislocations, postoperative disease, spondylolisthesis, fluorosis, Paget's disease[51] (Fig. 7), acromegaly, ankylosing spondylitis, calcification of the posterior longitudinal ligament[32,41] (Fig. 8), and thickening of ligamentum flavum with or without ossification.[47]

CT is particularly valuable in evaluation of lumbar spinal stenosis.[20] It is occasionally difficult to evaluate the upper thoracic and lower cervical spine due to the artifacts produced from the shoulders and the paucity of the epidural fat; however, the bony configuration and dimensions of the bony spinal canal can be accurately evaluated. The relationship of the thecal sac to the bony spinal canal should also be evaluated. The absence of epidural fat in suspected spinal stenosis suggests that clinically significant stenosis is present.[27]

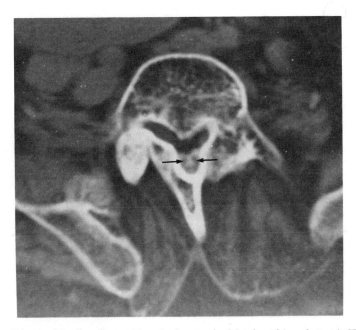

FIG 4. Diastrophic dwarfism with spinal stenosis. Metrizamide-enhanced CT scan at L5 shows severe narrowing of the spinal canal and small amount of metrizamide in the posterior spinal canal with demonstration of thickening of the nerve roots (black arrows) and absence of dorsal epidural fat.

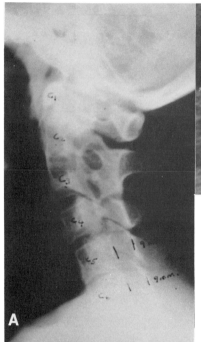

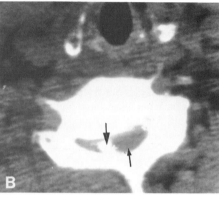

FIG 5. Klippel-Feil syndrome associated with spinal stenosis. *A*, Lateral cervical spinal film shows a fusion of C2 and C3 vertebrae and a narrow midsagittal spinal canal (9 mm at C5 and C6). *B*, Metrizamide-enhanced CT at C6 shows distortion of the thecal sac (black arrow), flattening and eccentric position of the cord (thin black arrow) due to a marked narrowing of sagittal spinal canal.

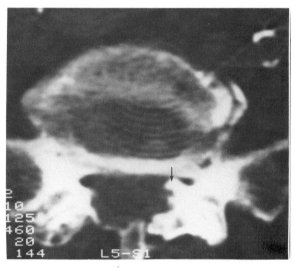

FIG 6. Severe degenerative disease and hypertrophy of the facet joints. CT at L5-S1 shows hypertrophic change (black arrow), particularly on the left side, which caused lateral recess stenosis. Subchondral cysts, sclerosis, and loss of cartilage involving bilateral facet joints are also seen.

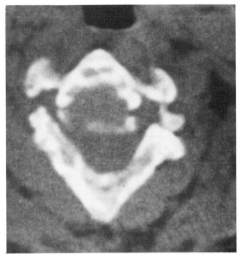

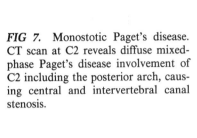

FIG 7. Monostotic Paget's disease. CT scan at C2 reveals diffuse mixed-phase Paget's disease involvement of C2 including the posterior arch, causing central and intervertebral canal stenosis.

Degenerative Diseases

Thickening of the Ligamenta Flava. The ligamenta flava are composed mainly of elastic connective tissues in a longitudinal array extending from the anterior inferior aspect of the lamina above a disc space to the posterior superior surface of the lamina below the disc space. Each half of the ligamentum flavum extends laterally from the midline to the intervertebral foramen, forming the posterior boundary and roof of the foramen. The ligaments then turn dorsally outside the foramina and fuse with the capsules of the articular facets. The thickness of the ligamentum flavum gradually increases from the cervical to the lumbar regions (1.5 mm at C2–C3 level;, 2.0 mm at T11–T12 and 4–6 mm in the lower lumbar spine). Thickening of ligamentum flavum is believed to be a

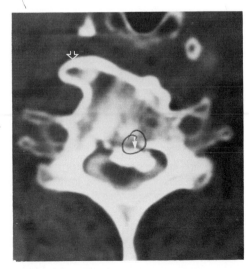

FIG 8. DISH (diffuse idiopathic skeletal hyperostosis) with spinal stenosis due to calcification of posterior longitudinal ligament. Intrathecal metrizamide-enhanced CT scan at C5 shows dense calcification of the posterior longitudinal ligament (white arrow) compressing the spinal cord and extensive osteophytosis (white open arrow) consistent with the diagnosis of DISH. Up to 25% of patients with DISH have calcification in the posterior longitudinal ligament.

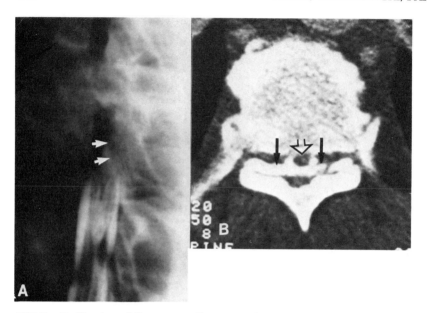

FIG 9.   Ossification of ligamentum flavum causing spinal stenosis and myelopathy. *A,* Lateral view of metrizamide myelogram shows complete block at lower T8 level produced by an extradural mass (white arrows). *B,* CT myelogram at T8-T9 level shows ossification of ligamentum flavum (arrows), small cord (open arrow), and spinal stenosis. Decompressive laminectomy at T8, T9, and T10 levels relieved clinical symptoms of spinal cord compression.

degenerative process produced by an increase in the amount of fibrous tissue. It is commonly associated with facet-joint degeneration.[47] It may also be a primary cause of spinal cord, cauda equina, or nerve-root symptoms.[8,36,38,47] Myelogram, CT myelogram (Fig. 9), and MRI (Fig. 10) may add more information as to the clinical significance of the disease.[18,39,47] The identification of facet joint disease or calcification of the ligamentum flavum is more efficient with CT scan than with MRI.[21] MRI with a GRASS (gradient recalled acquisition in the steady state) sequence shows a higher signal intensity for CSF compared with that of the spinal cord and extradural structures,[39] which may provide a rapid noninvasive study for spinal cord or thecal sac compression (Fig. 10B).

Degenerative Facet Disease and Synovial Cyst.   Facet joint arthropathy is not clearly demonstrated by plain films. CT readily visualizes the facet joints and can distinguish facet joint disease from disc disease. The combination of degenerative facet disease, thickening of ligamenta flava and generalized bulging disk is not unusual and may produce spinal stenosis (Fig. 11). Subchondral cysts, sclerosis, narrowing of joint space, osteophyte formations, vacuum phenomenon, and hypertrophy are seen in the articular facets in degenerative disease.[7] Spondylolisthesis without spondylolysis (Fig. 12) can be due to degenerative changes.

Synovial cyst is a cystic lesion of the synovial membrane which may or may not have a detectable pedicle attached to a synovial sheath or joint capsule

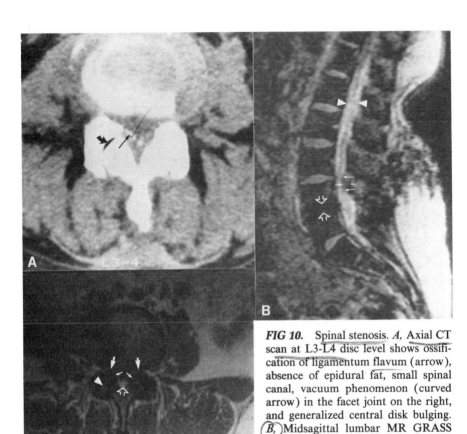

FIG 10. Spinal stenosis. *A,* Axial CT scan at L3-L4 disc level shows ossification of ligamentum flavum (arrow), absence of epidural fat, small spinal canal, vacuum phenomenon (curved arrow) in the facet joint on the right, and generalized central disk bulging. *B,* Midsagittal lumbar MR GRASS (gradient recalled acquisition in the steady state sequence) image (33/20, flip angles = 5°) shows extrinsic compression on the dorsal thecal sac (white arrows) by the thickened ligamentum flavum (small white arrows) at the L3-L4 level. Low-signal intensity (open white arrows) is seen at L4-L5 disc representing degenerative disc disease without focal herniation. Higher signal intensity (white arrow heads) in the spinal canal represents normal CSF flow. *C,* T1-weighted axial MR image (SE 1000/30) at L3-L4 disc level shows thickening of ligamenta flava (white arrows), generalized bulging disc (large white arrows), and low-signal intensity in the facet joint on the right representing vacuum phenomenon (white arrow head). Small amount of dorsal epidural fat (open white arrow) is seen as high-signal intensity, which is not seen on CT scan.

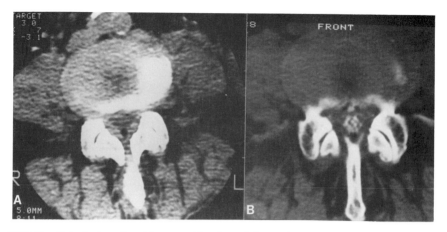

FIG 11. Spinal stenosis with a combination of facet disease, thickening of ligamenta flava, and generalized disc bulging. *A,* Axial plain CT, *B,* Axial CT myelogram at L4-L5 disc level reveals degenerative facet disease including narrowing of facet joint, osteophyte formation and sclerosis of the cortex of the facet processes, thickening of ligamenta flava, and bulging disc. The thecal sac is small and irregular due to extradural compression.

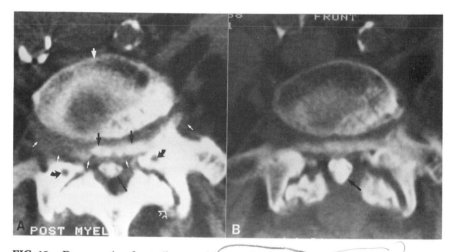

FIG 12. Degenerative facet disease with spondylolisthesis and spinal stenosis. *A,* Intrathecal metrizamide-enhanced CT scan at L5-S1 disc level shows posterior pseudo-bulging disk (white arrows), superior endplate of S1 (black arrows), lower endplate of L5 (large white arrow), subchondral cysts (black curved arrows), and osteophyte formation (white open arrow) of the facet, narrowing of the facet joints, and spinal stenosis with small and irregular thecal sac (large black arrow). *B,* Postoperative intrathecal metrizamide-enhanced axial CT scan at L5-S1 disc level shows posterior decompression with laminectomy and the thecal sac (black arrow) to be bigger and smoother than preoperatively.

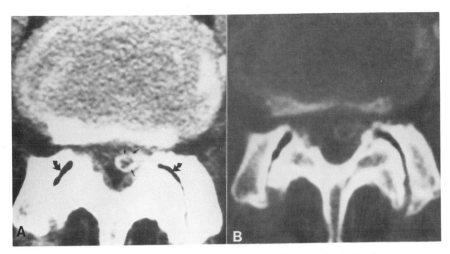

FIG 13. Synovial cyst of the lumbar spine with calcified wall. Axial CT scan at the level of L4-L5. Soft tissue setting (A) and bone setting (B) shows a synovial cyst with calcified wall (arrows) in the spinal canal adjacent to the facet capsule on the left. Degenerative facet disease is seen bilaterally including vacuum phenomenon (black curved arrows), sclerosis, osteophyte formation, and hypertrophy of the facet.

and which is filled with clear mucinous matter or gas.[22,46,49] It is caused by facet joint degeneration or herniation of synovium through the tears in the joint capsule. The most common site of these cysts is the L4–L5 facet-joint. CT scan is more reliable in making the diagnosis preoperatively. CT findings of a cyst lesion with calcified wall (Fig. 13) or a gas-filled cystic mass (Fig. 14) in the spinal canal adjacent to the facet-joints are relatively specific for a synovial cyst.

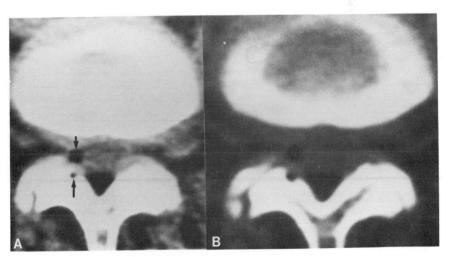

FIG 14. Synovial cyst of the lumbar spine with air in the cyst. Axial CT scan at L4-L5 level. Soft tissue setting (A) and bone setting (B) shows gas collection (arrow) in the synovial cyst on the right. Gas is also seen underneath the ligamentum flavum (large arrow). Degenerative facet disease is also seen, including narrowing of the joint space, sclerosis, osteophyte formation, and hypertrophy of the facet.

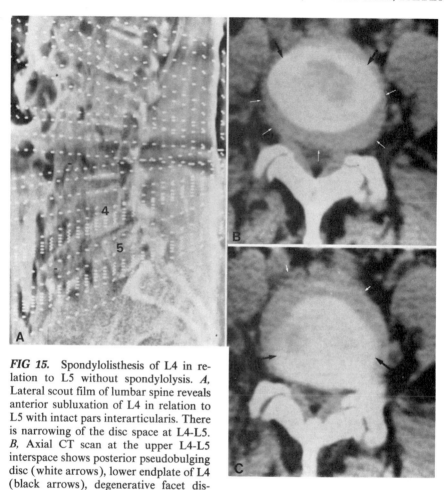

FIG 15. Spondylolisthesis of L4 in relation to L5 without spondylolysis. *A,* Lateral scout film of lumbar spine reveals anterior subluxation of L4 in relation to L5 with intact pars interarticularis. There is narrowing of the disc space at L4-L5. *B,* Axial CT scan at the upper L4-L5 interspace shows posterior pseudobulging disc (white arrows), lower endplate of L4 (black arrows), degenerative facet disease, thickening of ligamenta flava, and spinal stenosis. *C,* Axial CT scan at the lower L4-L5 interspace shows anterior pseudobulging disc (white arrows), upper endplate of L5 (black arrows), degenerative facet disease, thickening of ligamenta flava, and spinal stenosis.

SPONDYLOLISTHESIS AND SPONDYLOLYSIS

Spondylolisthesis is a condition in which one vertebra has slipped in relation to its next lower vertebra. This subluxation may be seen in the patients with a defect in the pars interarticularis but may also be seen in the patients with an intact pars interarticularis. Spondylolisthesis may be classified into six categories: dysplastic, isthmic, degenerative, traumatic, pathologic, or iatrogenic.[50]

Spondylolysis is a condition in which there is a presence of a fibrous cleft within the pars interarticularis that divides the vertebral arch into two segments:

the anterosuperior segment, consisting of the pedicle, the transvers
and the superior facet; and the posteroinferior segment, consisting of tl
spinous process, and the inferior facet. Spondylolysis occurs in 5% of tl
population.[42] Common sites of occurrence are at the levels of L5 (6
L4 (30%). The defects usually involve the pars interarticularis bilaterally. The
etiology of spondylolysis is uncertain; the most popular theory is that it results
from stress fractures of pars interarticularis due to repeated minor trauma.[50]

CT scan provides excellent information regarding bony abnormality and
soft tissue pathology. Sagittal and multiplanar reformatted images may provide
better delineation of bony pathology. Axial CT scan demonstrates a "double
canal" or "pseudo-bulging disc" appearance in spondylolisthesis as the vertebral
bodies become subluxed (Figs. 12, 15),[19] and shows an "incomplete posterior
ring" appearance in spondylolysis (Fig. 16).

TUMORS

High-resolution CT of the spine can be used reliably to visualize cortical
bone destruction, calcified tumor matrix, and soft tissue mass in the patient
with tumor involving the posterior spinal structures. However, accurate delineation in the anatomic relationships of the tumors, including bone involvement,
spinal canal or thecal sac invasion, and paraspinal soft-tissue extension sometimes
cannot be obtained without intrathecal introduction of nonionic water-soluble
contrast agents.[4,30] MRI can provide similar information to an intrathecal contrast-enhanced CT scan but is a noninvasive way to evaluate tumor involvement.[4]
Plain CT is superior to MRI in showing cortical bone destruction and calcified
tumor.

CT-guided percutaneous spinal biopsy can be performed safely and precisely
on an outpatient basis (Fig. 17).[23] A brief discussion of some various tumor
types involving the posterior spinal structures follows.

Osteoid Osteoma

Osteoid osteoma is a primary benign tumor of bone which comprises 11%
of all benign bone tumors, with spinal osteoid osteoma representing about 6%
of all benign bone tumors.[10] It affects males three times more often than females
and occurs most often in early adulthood. The most common location of the
lesion is the lumbar vertebrae (59%) (Fig. 18), followed by the cervical (27%)
(Fig. 19), thoracic (12%), and sacral (2%) vertebrae. The tumor most often
involves the neural arch (75%), particularly laminae (33%), articular facets
(9%), and pedicles (15%). The typical clinical presentation is that of back pain
that worsens at night and is relieved by aspirin. Mild scoliosis is often present.
The characteristic CT appearance of osteoid osteoma is: (1) a well-defined round
or oval low-density lesion (nidus), (2) high density in the center of the nidus
(mineralized osteoid, often misnamed sequestrum), and (3) various degrees of
surrounding reactive bone changes.[15]

Aneurysmal Bone Cyst

Aneurysmal bone cyst is an expansile cystic lesion of unknown etiology.
Most patients affected are under 20 years of age.[10] Only one quarter of aneurysmal

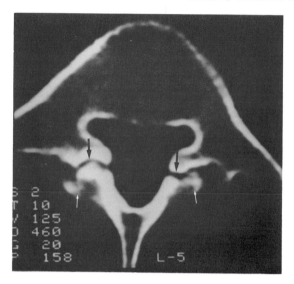

FIG 16. Axial CT scan with bone setting at L5 level shows defect at pars interarticularis (black arrows) (incomplete posterior ring) bilaterally. Osteophyte formations (white arrows) are seen adjacent to the bone defects at pars interarticularis.

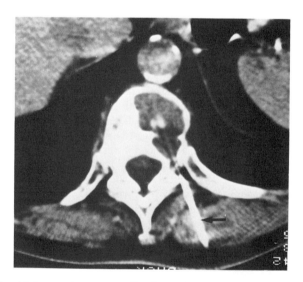

FIG 17. CT-guided percutaneous needle (arrow) aspiration biopsy of the osteolytic lesion of the pedicle of T7 on the left was performed under local anesthesia on an outpatient basis. Osteolytic bony destruction was also seen involving the vertebral body of T7 on the left. Pathologic diagnosis was metastatic breast carcinoma. Histologically, the biopsy specimen was identical to the surgical specimen of the breast resected 10 years ago.

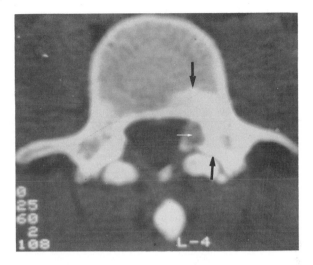

FIG 18. Osteoid osteoma of pedicle of L4. Axial CT scan shows a slight expansile lesion containing a calcification (white arrow) in the center of the low density nidus at the medial aspect of the pedicle of L4 on the left with surrounding reactive bone changes of dense sclerosis involving the pedicle and posterior vertebral body (black arrows).

bone cysts involve the spine or sacrum. The cervical and thoracic regions are the predominant sites of spinal involvement. Aneurysmal bone cysts primarily involve the posterior spinal bone elements and may expand into the pedicles and vertebral body. Pathologically, the lesions are composed of large fibrous-walled communicating cavities filled with unclotted blood. The differential diagnosis should include giant cell tumor and osteoblastoma. Plain spine film or CT scan shows expansile cystic lesion with an eggshell-like peripheral calcification. Myelogram may show the thecal sac and/or spinal cord compression (Fig. 20A). Intrathecal contrast-enhanced CT scan may reveal expansile bone changes, soft tissue mass, and spinal cord compression (Fig. 20B). Selective

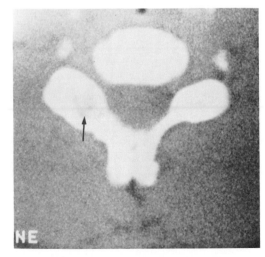

FIG 19. Osteoid osteoma of lamina of C5. Axial CT at C5 shows a discrete low density nidus (black arrow) surrounded by dense sclerotic hypertrophy of lamina of C5 on the right.

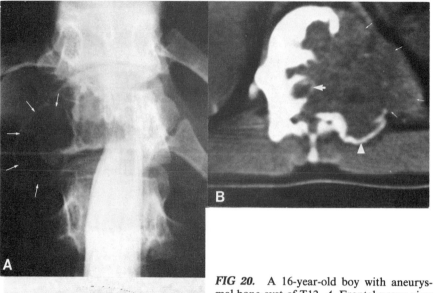

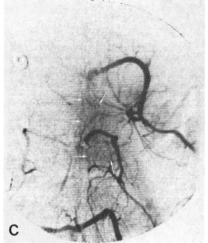

FIG 20. A 16-year-old boy with aneurysmal bone cyst of T12. *A,* Frontal prone view of metrizamide myelogram shows high-grade block of rostral flow and displacement of the spinal cord to the right at T12. A large expansile lytic lesion with eggshell-like peripheral calcification (white arrows) is seen at T12 on the left. *B,* Axial intrathecal metrizamide-enhanced CT at T12 shows lytic expansile lesion involving pedicle, lamina, and posterior vertebral body on the left with intraspinal and paraspinal soft tissue mass extension (white arrows). The spinal cord and thecal sac (large white arrow) are displaced to the right. Eggshell-like peripheral calcification (white arrowhead) is seen. *C,* Spinal DSA (digital subtraction arteriogram) shows tumor blush (white arrows). Anterior radiculomedullary arteries are identified several segments away from the mass.

spinal angiography (Fig. 20C) is used to identify the relationships of the feeding arteries, the anterior radiculomedullary artery, the artery of the Adamkiewicz, and the anterior spinal artery, and to assist the surgeon in operative planning.

Osteochondroma

Osteochondroma is a benign primary tumor consisting of cortical and trabecular bone covered with a cartilaginous cap of varying thickness. Hereditary multiple osteochondromas are a relatively common form of bone dysplasia, but lesions involving spine are rare. Solitary spinal osteochondromas are very rare, with one half of the reported cases located in the cervical spine.[24,29] Plain CT scan (Fig. 21) and CT scan with intrathecal contrast injection can demonstrate

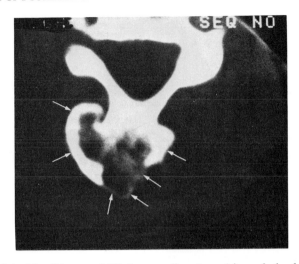

FIG 21. Axial plain CT scan of C5 shows a discrete and irregularly shaped expansile lesion involving the spinous process (white arrows) with dense bone and cartilage. The lesion was excised and the diagnosis was benign osteochondroma.

bony abnormality and neural foramina involvement and can visualize its extension in the spinal canal.

Metastases

Metastatic tumors of vertebrae, epidural masses, and paravertebral soft tissue masses can be accurately evaluated by high resolution CT scan.[48] Intrathecal contrast-enhanced CT provides better delineation of the relationship between the spinal cord and the metastases (Fig. 22).

FIG 22. Metastatic breast carcinoma. Axial CT scan at T11 with intrathecal contrast injection reveals lytic bone destruction involving spinal process (white arrows) and soft tissue mass compromising the dorsal spinal canal and displaced the spinal cord anteriorly.

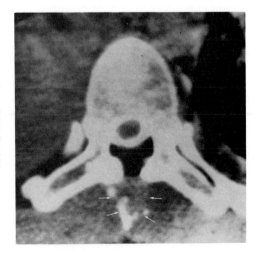

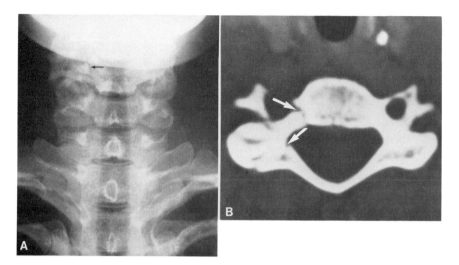

FIG 23. Comminuted fracture of C5 pedicle. *A,* Frontal view of plain film of cervical spine reveals a vertical radiolucent line through the pedicle of C5 on the right representing a fracture (arrow). *B,* Axial CT at C5 (bone setting) shows comminuted fracture of pedicle of C5 on right (white arrows) extending to the transverse process. The fracture is better delineated on CT than plain film. No bony fragment is seen projecting into the spinal canal.

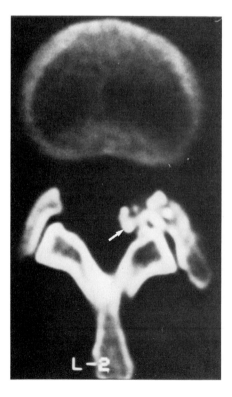

FIG 24. Axial CT at L2 shows comminuted fracture of superior articular facet on the left with retention of foreign body (white arrow) (small bullet fragments).

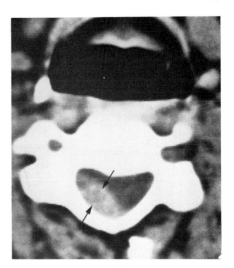

FIG 25. Axial CT scan at C5 shows high-density (55 Hounsfield units) epidural hematoma (arrows).

TRAUMA

The treatment and ultimate prognosis of spinal trauma are largely dependent on the accurate assessment of the precise level, anatomic location, and type of pathology. CT is easily obtained and has significantly aided the accurate diagnosis of spinal trauma.[13] Fracture of the neural arch and presence of bony fragment projecting into the spinal canal are more easily demonstrated on CT than on plain film or linear tomography (Fig. 23).[25] Associated paraspinal masses and related lesions are also better visualized on CT scan than plain film. Retention of foreign body (Fig. 24), disc herniation, intraspinal hematoma (Fig. 25), and the narrowing of the spinal canal or neural foramen can also be well identified on CT scan. Sagittal reformatted CT scan (Fig. 26) and CT with 3-D recon-

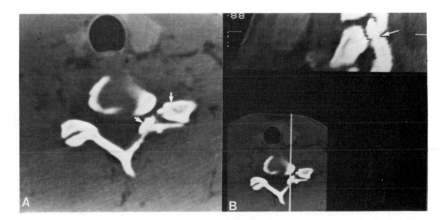

FIG 26. Fracture and subluxation of superior articular facet of C7 on the left. *A,* Axial CT scan at C6-C7 shows anterior subluxation of the fractured superior articular facet of C7 on the left (white arrows). *B,* Sagittal reformatted CT image shows fracture of the superior facet (white arrows) of C7 on the left, which is better defined on the reformatted image.

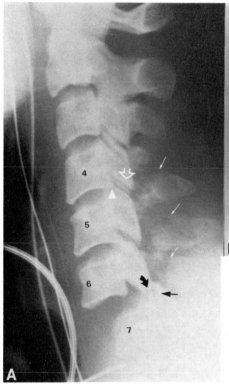

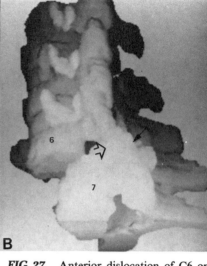

FIG 27. Anterior dislocation of C6 on C7. *A*, Lateral view of plain film of cervical spine shows anterior dislocation of C6 on C7 and fractures of the spinous process of C4, C5 and C6 (white arrows). There is locking facet of C6-C7 bilaterally. The inferior articular facet of C6 (curved black arrow) is anterior to the superior articular facet of C7 (black arrow). The normal superior articular facet (white arrow head) should be anterior to the inferior articular facet (white open arrow). Severe prevertebral soft tissue swelling is also seen. *B*, A 3-D reconstructed CT image shows anterior dislocation of C6 on C7 and locking facet of C6 (open arrow) and C7 (black arrow).

struction (Fig. 27) display bone anatomy and thus are useful in the diagnosis of fracture and dislocation of posterior spinal elements.

CONGENITAL ANOMALY
Absent Cervical Pedicle

Congenital absence of a cervical pedicle is a rare developmental anomaly that may present problems in the interpretation of plain film of cervical spine, particularly in the case of the symptomatic patient following trauma. Failure of diagnosing this abnormality correctly may lead to improper management. When absence of a pedicle with enlargement of the neural foramen is found on plain film, differential diagnosis includes fracture and subluxation, osteolytic metastasis, primary bone tumor, and neurogenic tumor. Familiarity with the characteristic CT features of absent cervical pedicle and identification of the intact cortex of the adjacent bone may provide great help to avoid improper treatment (Fig. 28).

The vertebra develops from six centers of chondrification: two for the vertebral body; two for the pedicles, lateral masses, and dorsal transverse proc-

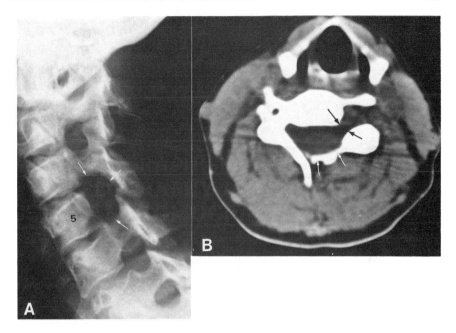

FIG 28. Congenital absence of cervical pedicle. A 40-year-old female with mild neck pain following a motor vehicle accident. *A,* Oblique view of cervical spine reveals absence of the pedicle on C5 on the left resulting in apparently enlargement of neural foramen (white arrows). *B,* Axial CT at C5 shows absence of pedicle on the left (black arrows) and hypoplasia of the lamina on the left (white arrows). The bone cortex is intact.

esses; and two for the lamina and spinous process. The embryologic basis for congenital absence of a pedicle is the lack of development of the vertebral chondrification centers, which are responsible for forming the pedicle, the dorsal part of the transverse process, and the lateral mass.[9] The characteristic CT findings of congenital absence of a cervical pedicle are: (1) complete absence of the involved pedicle, (2) widening of the intervertebral foramen, (3) dorsal displacement of the lateral mass, (4) well-defined cortex of the adjacent bone, (5) absence of the dorsal portion of the transverse process with excessive length or angulation of the remaining ventral portion, and (6) straight posterior border of the affected vertebral body.[9]

Spina Bifida, Meningocele, Myelomeningocele, Lipomyelomeningocele

Spina bifida is a dysraphism of osseous elements that form to close the spinal canal. Spina bifida aperta (or spina bifida cystica) implies a herniation of all or part of the spinal contents through a posterior spina bifida to form an obvious protrusion. Spina bifida occulta is a group of spinal dysraphisms without obvious cystic mass.

Meningocele is a form of spina bifida aperta with a midline, skin-covered protrusion of dura and arachnoid through a spinal defect into the subcutaneous tissue of the back.

Myelomeningocele is a form of spina bifida aperta with a midline neural

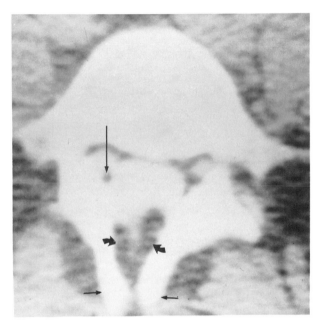

FIG 29.   Spina bifida aperta. Axial CT scan at L5 following myelogram shows nonfused spinous process (black arrows), tethering cord (long black arrow), and lipoma (curved black arrows).

tissue protrusion elevated above the skin surface of the back by expansion of the subarachnoid space ventral to the cord and neural plaque. Lipoma may be associated with either meningocele or myelomeningocele.

CT scan with intrathecal contrast injection can clearly demonstrate tethering spinal cord, meningocele, lipoma, and posterior spinal fusion defect (Fig. 29). High-resolution MRI of the spine can be used effectively in the noninvasive evaluation of patients with congenital spinal anomaly, spina bifida aperta, or lipomyelomeningocele (Fig. 30).[21]

INFECTION

CT manifestations of spinal infection include paravertebral soft tissue swelling, abscess formation, and bone erosion.[17] The main advantage of CT is exquisite sensitivity to soft tissue and bony abnormalities. The early stages of spinal infection in paravertebral abscess, epidural abscess, and spinal cord compression are more likely to be diagnosed with CT than with conventional radiography. CT-guided percutaneous aspiration biopsy can be performed safely and precisely. Spinal epidural abscess may be acute or chronic. Acute abscess tends to appear in the spinal epidural space initially, either as a result of bacteremia or a primary local infection. CT scan with intrathecal contrast injection via a C1-C2 puncture may delineate the extension of the epidural abscess, the thecal sac, or spinal cord displacement (Fig. 31). MRI may provide similar information on a noninvasive basis.[34] Epidural abscess associated with vertebral osteomyelitis is more likely to be chronic and may be diagnosed accurately by plain spinal CT scan.

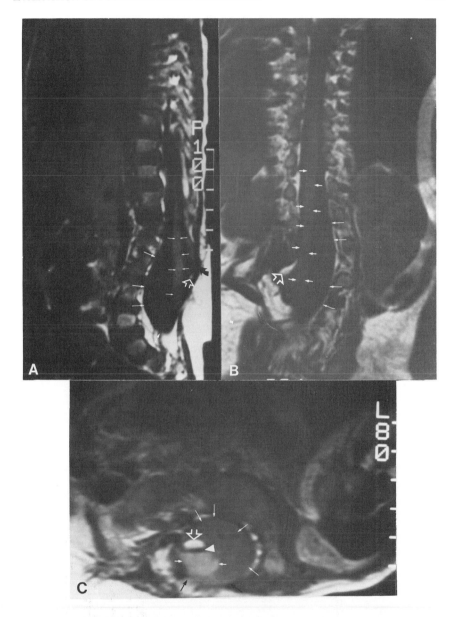

FIG 30. Spina bifida aperta with lipomyelomeningocele. *A,* Midsagittal T1-weighted MR image (SE 500/20) of thoracolumbosacral spine demonstrates tethering cord (white arrows), enlarged thecal sac (large white arrows), lipoma (open white arrows), and meningocele (black curved arrow) at lower lumbar region. *B,* Coronal T1-weighted MR image (SE 400/20) of thoracolumbosacral spine demonstrates tethering cord (white arrows), enlarged thecal sac (large white arrows), and lipoma (white open arrow). *C,* Axial proton density weighted (SE 2000/30) image at level of L5 shows spina bifida (black arrows), enlarged thecal sac (large white arrows), tethering cord (small white arrows), lipoma (open white arrow), and chemical shift artifact (white arrow head).

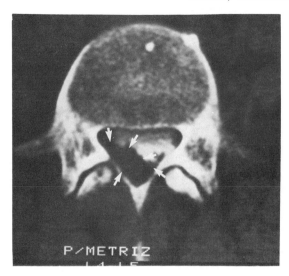

FIG 31. A 21-year-old male with heroin addiction presented with back pain and fever. CT scan at L4 level with intrathecal injection of metrizamide via a lateral C1-C2 approach showed epidural abscess (white arrows) on the right which displaced the thecal sac anteriorly and to the left side. The abscess was drained and the culture was *Staphylococcus aureus.*

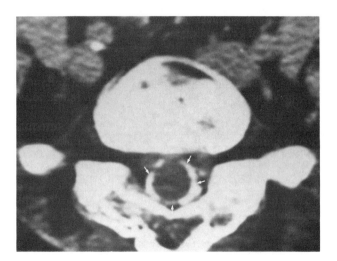

FIG 32. Arachnoiditis ossificans. Axial CT at L5-S1 level shows a calcified ring (white arrows) in the periphery of the thecal sac representing arachnoiditis ossificans. This is probably related to previous surgery of posterior spinal fusion.

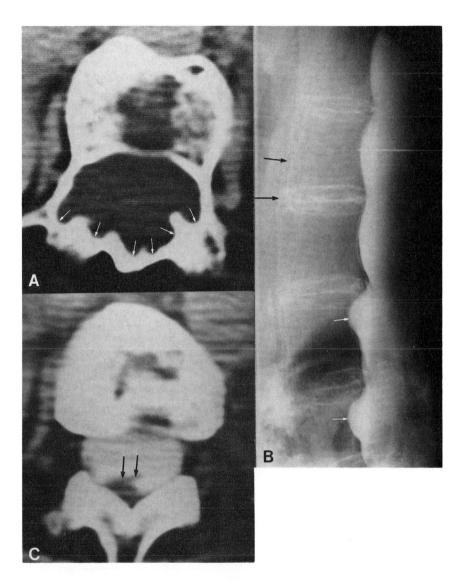

FIG 33.   Ankylosing spondylitis with cauda equina syndrome. *A,* Axial CT at L1 demonstrates marked lobulated expansion of the bony canal and erosion of the posterior bony spinal elements (white arrows). *B,* Lateral film of metrizamide myelogram shows complete bony bridge (black arrows) anteriorly across the lumbar vertebrae. There are dura ectasia and arachnoid diverticula (white arrows). *C,* Axial CT at L1-L2 interspace level following metrizamide myelogram shows irregular appearance of the thecal sac posteriorly (black arrows) and nonvisualization of the individual nerve roots consistent with arachnoiditis.

MISCELLANEOUS
Arachnoiditis Ossificans

Spinal arachnoiditis ossificans, which is due to degeneration of arachnoid cell clusters, presents as deposition of bone matrix within the inflamed arachnoid tissues. The etiologies are trauma, hemorrhage, previous myelogram, and spinal anesthesia. CT findings are concentric calcified rings (Fig. 32) surrounding the thecal sac or calcification surrounding the spinal cord.[37] Arachnoiditis ossificans is not reliably identified by MRI due to lack of signal from calcification.

Ankylosing Spondylitis with Cauda Equina Syndrome

This rare form of vertebral bone erosion is seen in patients with ankylosing spondylitis who develop cauda equina syndrome. CT scan shows lobulated bone expansion with erosion of the posterior spinal bony elements (Fig. 33A). On metrizamide myelogram and CT myelogram, there is an enlarged lobulated thecal sac (dural ectasia and diverticulum) with the appearance of arachnoiditis (Figs. 33B, C). Arachnoiditis with the formation of the arachnoid cysts and pulsatile expansion of arachnoid cysts may result in cauda equina syndrome.[6,43]

REFERENCES

1. Axel L: Surface coil magnetic resonance imaging. J Comput Assist Tomogr 8:381–384, 1984.
2. Badgley CE: Articular facets in relation to low back pain and sciatic radiation. J Bone Joint Surg 23:481–496, 1941.
3. Barnes PD, Lester PD, Yamanashi WS, Prince JR: Magnetic resonance imaging in infants and children with spinal dysraphism. AJNR 7:465–472, 1986.
4. Beltran J, Noto AM, Chakeres DW, Christoforidis AJ: Tumors of the osseous spine: staging with MR imagining versus CT. Radiology 162:565–569, 1987.
5. Bethem D, Winter RB, Lutter L: Disorders of the spine in diastrophic dwarfism. A discussion of nine patients and review of the literature. J Bone Joint Surg 62:529–536, 1986.
6. Byrne JV: Case of the season. Semin Roentgenol 21:101–102, 1986.
7. Carrera GF, Haughton VM, Syvertsen A, Williams AL: Computed tomography of the lumbar facet joints. Radiology 134:145–148, 1980.
8. Chintapalli K: Progressive myelopathy in a 32 year old man. JAMA 253:2255–2257, 1985.
9. Cox HE, Bennett WF: Computed tomography of absent cervical pedicle. J Comput Assist Tomogr 8:537–539, 1984.
10. Dahlin DC: Bone Tumors: General Aspects and Data on 6221 Cases, 3rd ed. Springfield, IL, Charles C Thomas, 1978
11. Epstein BS, Epstein JA, Jones MD: Cervical spinal stenosis. Radiol Clin North Am 15:215–226, 1977.
12. Epstein BS, Epstein JA, Jones MD: Lumbar spinal stenosis. Radiol Clin North Am 15:227–239, 1977.
13. Faerber EN, Wolpert SM, Scott RM, et al: Computed tomography of spinal fractures. J Comput Assist Tomogr 3:657–661, 1979.
14. Freiherr G: 3-D imaging in medicine: synthesizing the third dimension. Diagn Imag 11:190–203, 1987.
15. Gamba JL, Martinez S, Apple J, et al: Computed tomography of axial skeletal osteoid osteomas. AJR 142:769–772, 1984.
16. Glenn WV, Jr., Rhodes ML, Altschuler EM, et al: Multiplanar display computerized body tomography applications in the lumbar spine. Spine 4:282–352, 1979.
17. Golimbu C, Firooznia H, Rafii M: CT of osteomyelitis of the spine. AJR 142:159–163, 1984.
18. Grenier N, Kressel HY, Schiebler ML, et al: Normal and degenerative posterior spinal structures: MR imaging. Radiology 165:517–525, 1987.
19. Grogan JP, Heminghytt S, Williams AL, et al: Spondylolysis studied with computed tomography. Radiology 145:737–742, 1982.
20. Hammerschlag SB, Wolpert SM, Carter BL: Computed tomography of the spinal canal. Radiology 121:361–367, 1976.
21. Haughton VM: MR imaging of the spine. Radiology 166:297–301, 1988.

22. Hemminghytt S, Daniels DL, Williams AL, Haughton VM: Intraspinal synovial cysts: Nature, history and diagnosis by CT. Radiology 145:375–376, 1982.

23. Herkowitz HN, Wesolowski DP: Percutaneous biopsy of the spine: indications, techniques, results, and complications. Update on Spinal Disorders 1:3–9, 1986.

24. Julien J, Riemens V, Vital C, Lagueny A: Cervical cord compression by solitary osteochondroma of the atlas. J Neurol Neurosurg Psychiatry 41:479–481, 1978.

25. Kershner MS, Goodman GA, Perlmutter GS: Computed tomography in the diagnosis of an atlas fracture. Am J Roentgenol 128:688–689, 1977.

26. Kilcoyne RF, Mark LA: Computed tomography of spinal fractures. Appl Radiol 16:40–54, 1987.

27. Kirkhaldy-Willis WH, Paine KWE, et al: Lumbar spinal stenosis. Clin Orthop 99:30–50, 1974.

28. Langston JW, Gravant ML: "Incomplete ring" sign: a simple method for CT detection of spondylolysis. J Comput Assist Tomogr 9:728–729, 1985.

29. Lanzieri CF, Solodnik P, Sacher M, Herman G: Computed tomography of solitary spinal osteochondromas. J Comput Assist Tomogr 9:1042–1044, 1985.

30. Lee BCP, Kazam E, Newman AD: Computed tomography of the spine and spinal cord. Radiology 128:95–102, 1978.

31. Maslow GS, Rothman R: The facet joints: another look. Bull NY Acad Med 51:1294–1311, 1975.

32. Minagi H, Gronner AT: Calcification of the posterior longitudinal ligament: a cause of cervical myelopathy. Am J Roentgenol 105:365–369, 1969.

33. Modic MT, Feiglin DH, Piraino DW, et al: Vertebral osteomyelitis: assessment using MR. Radiology 157:157–166, 1985.

34. Modic MT, Masaryk T, Boomphrey F, et al: Lumbar herniated disc and canal stenosis: prospective evaluation by surface coil MR, CT and myelography. AJNR 7:709–717, 1986.

35. Mooney V, Robertson J: The facet syndrome. Clin Orthop 115:149–156, 1976.

36. Miyasaka K, Kiyoshi K, Ito T, et al: Ossification of spinal ligaments causing thoracic radiculomyelopathy. Radiology 143:463–468, 1982.

37. Nainkin L: Arachnoiditis ossificans. Report of a case. Spine 3:83–86, 1978.

38. Omojola MF, Cardosa ER, Fox AJ, et al: Thoracic myelopathy secondary to ossified ligamentum flavum. J Neurosurg 56:448–450, 1982.

39. Perkins TG, Wehrli FW: CSF signal enhancement in short TR gradient echo images. Magn Reson Imag 4:465–467, 1986.

40. Prusick VR, Samberg LC, Wesolowski DP: Klippel-Feil syndrome associated with spinal stenosis. A case report. J Bone Joint Surg 67:161–164, 1985.

41. Resnick D, Guerra J, Jr., Robinson CA, Vint VC: Association of diffuse idiopathic skeletal hyperostosis (DISH) and calcification of the posterior longitudinal ligament. AJR 131:1049–1053, 1978.

42. Roche MB, Rowe GG: The incidence of separate neural arch and coincident bone variations. A survey of 4200 skeletons. Anat Rec 109:233–259, 1951.

43. Rosenkranz W: Ankylosing spondylitis: cauda equina syndrome with multiple spinal cysts. Case report. J Neurosurg 34:241–243, 1971.

44. Rothman SLG, Glenn WV Jr.: CT multiplanar reconstruction in 253 cases of lumbar spondylolisthesis. AJNR 5:81–90, 1984.

45. Schellinger D, Wener L, Ragsdale BP, Patronas NJ: Facet joint disorders and their role in the production of back pain and sciatica. Radiographics 7:923–944, 1987.

46. Schulz EE, West WL, Hinshaw DB, Johnson DR: Gas in lumbar extradural juxtaarticular cyst: sign of synovial origin. Am J Roentgenol 143:875–876, 1984.

47. Stollman A, Pinto R, Benjamin V, Kricheff I: Radiologic imaging of symptomatic ligamentum flavum thickening with and without ossification. AJNR 8:991–994, 1987.

48. Wang A-M, Lewis ML, Rumbaugh CL, et al: Spinal cord or nerve root compression in patients with malignant disease: CT evaluation. J Comput Assist Tomogr 8:420–428, 1984.

49. Wang A-M, Haykal HA, Lin J C-T, Lee J-H: Synovial cysts of the lumbar spine: CT evaluation. Comput Radiol 11:253–257, 1987.

50. Wiltze LL: The etiology of spondylolithesis. J Bone Joint Surg 44A:539–569, 1963.

51. Zlatkin MB, Lander PH, Hadjipavlou AG, Levine JS: Paget's disease of the spine: CT with clinical correlation. Radiology 160:155–159, 1986.

REBECCA AYRES, MD

SPINAL DYSRAPHISM: EVALUATION BY MYELOGRAPHY AND COMPUTED TOMOGRAPHY

From the Department of Radiology, Scottish Rite Children's Hospital, Atlanta, Georgia

Reprint requests to:
Rebecca Ayres, MD
Department of Radiology
Scottish Rite Children's Hospital
1001 Johnson Ferry Road, NE
Atlanta, GA 30363

Spinal dysraphism is the term Lichtenstein applied in 1940 to malformations resulting from the inadequate or improper fusion of the median tissues of the back.[23] The affected tissues may include the skin, subcutaneous soft tissues, spine, meninges, and spinal cord. Spinal dysraphism comprises disorders ranging in severity from spina bifida with widening of the dural sac to complex malformations such as myelomeningocele with hydromyelia and the Chiari malformation.

Several imaging modalities are now available for evaluating the patient with spinal dysraphism. Spine radiographs display the vertebral anomalies, and are particularly useful for defining abnormalities of fusion and segmentation. Ultrasound, which is nonvasive and does not use ionizing radiation, can show fetal dysraphism in utero.[8,38] Ultrasound used postnatally can show abnormalities of the spinal cord and meninges where overlying spina bifida is present.[24,33] However, sonograms of the caudal spine may be difficult to interpret, and cannot be performed at those levels at which an intact neural arch prevents transmission of sound waves. Magnetic resonance imaging (MRI), which also does not use ionizing radiation, displays beautifully many of the abnormalities seen in spinal dysraphism.[2,19,21,30,31,36] However, in institutions where MRI is not available, and for patients in whom this scan is inconclusive or technically inadequate, myelography and computed tomography (CT) after intrathecal injection of water-soluble myelographic contrast medium continue to play the major role in evaluating the patient with spinal dysraphism.

A formal myelogram may be performed first, followed by a CT scan of those areas that appear abnormal or equivocal on the myelogram. Alternatively, a smaller dose of myelographic contrast material may be injected into the subarachnoid space and CT alone performed. Until recently, the myelographic contrast medium employed has been metrizamide, an ionic water-soluble compound. Newer non-ionic contrast material, such as iohexol, has an increased cost, but decreased incidence and severity of side effects.[20,28]

WIDENED THECAL SAC

A widened dural sac is the mildest form of this meningeal dysraphism.[29] Myelography and CT with myelographic contrast (CTM) show expansion of the spinal canal and thecal sac without an associated mass lesion or spinal cord abnormality.

TETHERED CORD

The tethered cord, also known as the filum terminale syndrome,[12] tight filum terminale,[16] and tethered conus,[11] is one of the commonest forms of spinal dysraphism. Patients present with various signs and symptoms, including sensorimotor deficit, bladder and bowel dysfunction, scoliosis, foot deformity, and low back pain.[13] About half of patients have cutaneous or subcutaneous abnormalities, such as hypertrichosis, lipomas, dermoids, and sinus tracts.[11]

The normal position of the conus ascends with age because of greater longitudinal growth of the spinal canal than the spinal cord. At three months of gestation, the spinal cord extends down to the coccyx.[32] At birth, the level of the conus ranges from L1 to L4, the average level being the lower border of L2.[3] Fitz and Harwood-Nash accept the L2–3 disc space as the lowermost

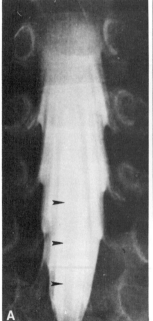
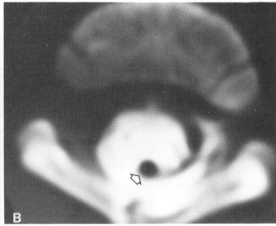

FIGURE 1. Tethered conus. *A*, Myelogram shows the tip of the conus at L3. Filum terminale (arrows) is abnormally thick. *B*, CTM image at L5 shows that filum is of the same low density as epidural fat, reflecting fatty infiltration of the filum.

normal position of the conus in infants.[11] By 12 years, the tip of the conus should lie at or above the mid L2 level. The normal filum terminale has a diameter of less than 2 mm.[11]

In the most subtle form of tethered cord, the conus lies slightly lower than normal and the filum is thickened, but no abnormal lipomatous tissue is present. In other cases, associated fatty tissue produces a diffusely thickened filum or expansion of the tip of the filum. Myelography cannot distinguish between filum that is thickened and that which is surrounded by lipomatous tissue, but CTM can distinguish the lower-density fat from the filum (Fig. 1). In the most severe form of tethered conus, the spinal cord extends into the lower lumbar or sacral region. The conus may not show its usual enlargement, the cord instead tapering gradually into a thickened tube. Most often, this tube represents spinal cord, and no true filum is present. In other cases, this tube is a filum surrounded by lipomatous tissue.[9] The cord can be distinguished from the filum on myelography by the emergence of nerve roots from the cord. The caudal nerve roots show an abnormally horizontal course when the cord is inferiorly positioned (Fig. 2).

MENINGOCELE, MYELOMENINGOCELE, AND LIPOMYELOMENINGOCELE

A meningocele is the protrusion of the meninges outside the spinal canal. A myelomeningocele is a meningocele that contains the spinal cord or nerve roots. A lipomyelomeningocele is a myelomeningocele containing lipomatous tissue.

The typical meningocele consists of a protrusion of dura and arachnoid posteriorly through a bifid neural arch. The spinal cord is tethered but does not

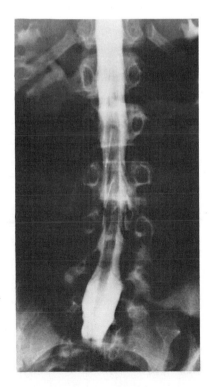

FIGURE 2. Tethered spinal cord. Spinal cord extends caudally to sacral tip of dural sac. Nerve roots exiting from the lumbar and sacral portions of the spinal cord course abnormally horizontally or even ascend toward the neural foramina.

protrude beyond the spinal canal.[10] Rarely, the meningocele may protrude anterior or laterally. The anterior sacral meningocele usually occurs at the sacral level. Plain films show an asymmetric sacral defect, which gives the sacrum a "scimitar" configuration.[9] Myelography and CTM demonstrate a collection of cerebrospinal fluid extending from the spinal canal through the defect into the pelvis.[35]

The myelomeningocele is five to ten times more common than the meningocele. Eighty to ninety percent of myelomeningoceles occur in the lower thoracic or lumbar spine, although the bony defect usually extends into the sacrum.[6] The spinal cord widens and flattens into a placode at the posterior margin of the myelomeningocele. The placode resembles a spinal cord that has been slit sagitally posteriorly and flattened out. The ventral nerve roots exit from the medial aspect of the placode, and the dorsal roots exit from the lateral edges.[10] Myelography and CTM show these nerve roots coursing anteriorly from the plaque into the spinal canal.

The myelomeningocele, unlike the meningocele and lipomyelomeningocele, is almost always associated with the Chiari II malformation of the lower brain stem and cerebellum.[10] Myelography and CTM show the inferiorly positioned cerebellar tonsils and medulla extending into the cervical spinal canal (Fig. 3).

The myelomeningocele is usually repaired shortly after birth without imaging studies. Myelography and CTM are usually done when the child is older because of the progression of neurologic symptoms. These studies frequently reveal tethering of the cord posteriorly at the site of surgery (Fig. 4).[14] They also show frequently associated lesions such as diastematomyelia and hydromyelia.

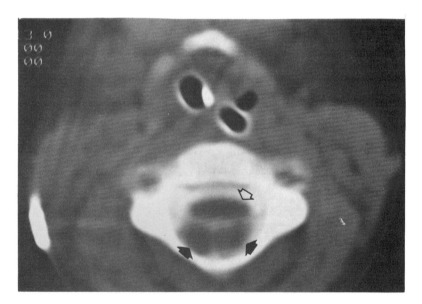

FIGURE 3. Chiari malformation. Cerebellar tonsils (solid arrows) extend into cervical spinal canal down to C4 level. The spinal cord (open arrow) anterior to the tonsils is flat, reflecting a collapsed hydromyelia. This is the same patient shown in Figure 9C, in whom the thoracolumbar portion of the hydromyelia is distended.

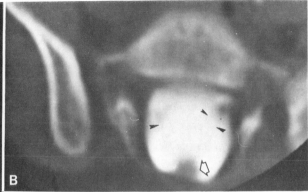

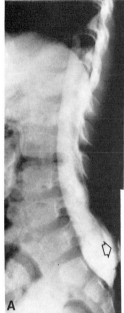

FIGURE 4. Repaired myelomeningocele. *A,* Four-year-old after repair of myelomeningocele at birth. A residual lumbosacral myelomeningocele is present. Spina bifida is present inferior to L2. At and superior to L3, a thin layer of opacified cerebrospinal fluid separates the posterior aspect of the spinal cord from the dural sac. At L4–5, the level of previous surgery, the repaired neural placode is adherent posteriorly to the dural sac. The neural tissue (open arrow) re-emerges into the thecal sac at S1. *B,* Three-year-old after myelomeningocele repair. CTM at sacral level shows the repaired neural placode (open arrow) adherent posteriorly to the dural sac. Nerve roots (arrows) course anteriorly into the subarachnoid space from the anterior aspect of the placode.

Lipomyelomeningoceles are about one-tenth as common as myelomeningoceles.[10] The patient usually has lumbosacral spina bifida with an overlying subcutaneous lipoma. The lipomatous tissue extends through the bifid neural arch and a dorsal defect in the dura, and becomes attached to the neural placode. This placode has the same anatomic arrangement as that in the myelomeningocele. A meningocele usually balloons posterolaterally around the neural placode and lipoma (Fig. 5). The lipoma may also extend into the spinal canal extradurally to form prominent fat pads around the thecal sac.[26]

DIASTEMATOMYELIA

Diastematomyelia is the partial or complete sagittal splitting of the spinal cord, conus medullaris, or filum terminale. This cleavage produces two hemicords, each of which contains one dorsal horn that gives rise to the ipsilateral dorsal nerve root, and one ventral horn that gives rise to the ipsilateral ventral nerve root. A bony or fibrous septum may extend through the split in the cord, but the diagnosis of diastematomyelia does not depend on the presence of such a septum.[25] In contrast to diastematomyelia is diplomyelia, which reflects complete duplication of the spinal cord. In this condition, each cord has its own dura and gives off two dorsal horns, two ventral horns, and four nerve roots at each level. Diplomyelia is seen with duplication of the spine, and is rarely diagnosed antemortem.[25]

Vertebral anomalies seen in diastematomyelia include spina bifida, fusion of vertebral bodies or neural arches, hemivertebrae, increased interpediculate

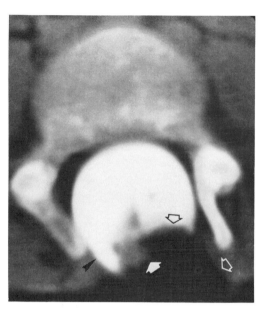

FIGURE 5. Lipomyelomeningocele. CTM at L4 level shows low-density fat (open black and white arrows) extending from the gluteal region through the spina bifida and a dorsal defect in the dura to merge with the neural placode (white solid arrow), which shows a higher density. A small meningocele (black arrows) protrudes posteriorly on the side opposite the bulk of the lipomatous tissue.

distance, and decreased anteroposterior diameter of vertebral bodies.[34] Scoliosis is present in over half of the cases.[15] A bony spur may be visible on plain radiographs, but can usually be seen more clearly on CT. Diastematomyelia is most common in the lower thoracic and upper lumbar regions, but cleavage of the cord may rarely occur as high as the cervical level.[15,22]

In at least one-half of the cases, no bony or fibrous septum is present. The spinal cord splits into two hemicords, both of which lie within a single arachnoid and dural tube (Fig. 6).[15,25,34] The hemicords may or may not reunite inferiorly. In the other type of diastematomyelia, a bony spur extends through the medullary cleft (Fig. 7). This septum splits the meninges as well as the cords, so that each hemicord is enclosed in its own dura and arachnoid at the level of the septum. Above and below the spur, the meninges reunite to form a single dural and arachnoid sheath. The length of the cleavage in the cord is necessarily longer than that of the split in the meninges. The hemicords may be symmetric or asymmetric in size, and usually reunite to form a single cord below the spur. In most cases of diastematomyelia, the spinal cord or hemicords are tethered.[15,25]

Myelography displays the defect in the thecal sac produced by a sagitally oriented spur but may fail to demonstrate an obliquely oriented spur.[9] Myelography frequently fails to show splitting of the spinal cord.[34] CTM more clearly shows the bony spur, the presence and extent of cleavage of the cord, and commissural bands joining the hemicords.[25]

HYDROMYELIA

Hydromyelia (congenital distention of the central canal of the spinal cord) and syringomyelia (cyst formation in the spinal cord outside the central canal) are difficult to distinguish radiographically, and the two entities may coexist. However, in the child with dysraphism, cavitation of the spinal cord usually indicates hydromyelia.[9]

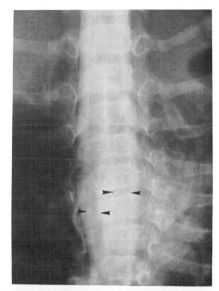

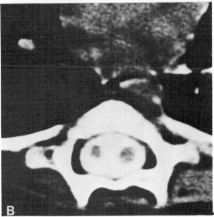

FIGURE 6. Diastematomyelia: single dural tube. *A,* Myelogram shows cleavage of spinal cord into two hemicords (arrows) from T5–T11. The hemicords are contained within a single dural sac. No spur is present between hemicords, which reunite at T12. The tip of the conus (not shown) lay at L3. Note widening of spinal canal and dural sac at the level of the diastematomyelia. *B,* CTM outlines the hemicords, asymmetric in size, and clearly defines the abnormal vertebral configuration.

Hydromyelia most frequently involves the cervical or upper thoracic chord but may extend throughout the cord.[29] When the hydromyelic cavity is distended, myelography and CTM show a rounded, enlarged cord (Fig. 8). When the cavity is collapsed, the cord appears flattened anteroposteriorly and slightly increased in transverse diameter (Fig. 3). The flattened cord is more common in children than is the expanded cord.[10] Kan et al. report a change in the anteroposterior diameter of the cord with changes in the patient's position during metrizamide myelography.[17]

Occasionally, the cavity is inadvertently punctured during myelography and the cyst itself is opacified. The hydromyelic cavity often shows irregular constrictions, giving a serrated contour to the dilated central canal (Fig. 9).[28] Computed tomographic images obtained from 6 to 24 hours after intrathecal contrast injection may show opacification of the hydromyelic cavity, either by

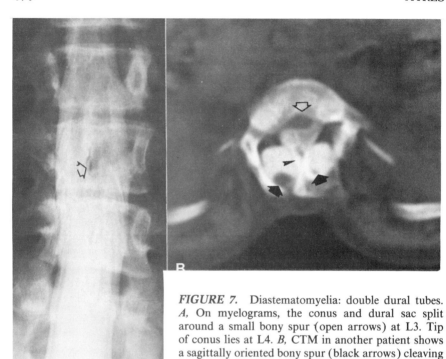

FIGURE 7. Diastematomyelia: double dural tubes. *A*, On myelograms, the conus and dural sac split around a small bony spur (open arrows) at L3. Tip of conus lies at L4. *B*, CTM in another patient shows a sagittally oriented bony spur (black arrows) cleaving the meninges and spinal cord to form two dural sacs and two hemicords (solid black arrows). A synchondrosis (open arrow) separates the vertebral body from the bony spur.

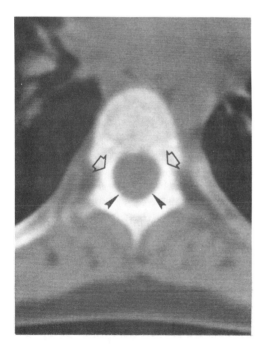

FIGURE 8. Hydromyelia. On CTM at T6, an enlarged rounded spinal cord (arrows) fills almost the entire spinal canal, leaving only a thin rim of opacified cerebrospinal fluid (open arrow).

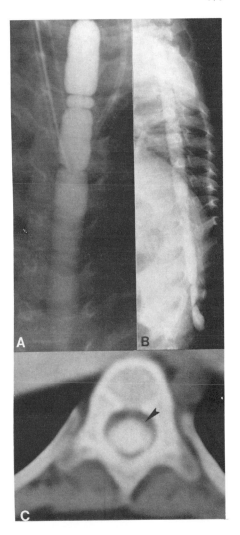

FIGURE 9. Hydromyelia. *A and B,* Four-year-old with repaired myelomeningocele. In an attempted myelogram, contrast was inadvertently injected into the hydromyelic cavity, which extends from C6 to L1. The patient had no apparent ill effects from the injection. PA view shows serrated contour of cephalic end of hydromyelic cavity. *C,* CTM in another patient shows myelographic contrast accidentally injected into the hydromyelic cavity (arrows). The surrounding spinal cord tissue is too thin to be detected on this image.

passage of contrast through a patent obex or diffusion through the cord itself.[1,18] This delayed opacification occurs in about one half of pediatric cases.[9]

As hydromyelia is frequently accompanied by Chiari malformation, the occipito-cervical junction warrants careful evaluation on metrizamide myelography and CTM for evidence of inferior tonsillar displacement.

NEURENTERIC CYST

At the third week of embryogenesis, the ectoderm (primitive neural tissue) and endoderm (primitive foregut) lie adjacent to each other. The neurenteric cyst, which is a cyst lined with gastrointestinal epithelium, is believed to arise from inadequate separation of the ectoderm and endoderm. Several theories attempt to explain this inadequate separation, including persistence of the neurenteric canal of Kovalevsky, splitting of the notochord, and failure of the notochord to separate the ectoderm and endoderm.[4,5,7,27,29,37] The most common configuration of the neurenteric cyst is an intraspinal cyst connected through a defect in the vertebral body to a prevertebral cyst. This lesion occurs most frequently at the cervicothoracic junction,[5] the prevertebral mass usually lying caudal to the vertebral defect. The anterior vertebral anomaly may range from a defect easily visible on plain films, such as a butterfly vertebra, to a tiny canal visible only on tomography or CT. As the prevertebral mass is typically in the posterior mediastinum, it is usually visible on plain films and CT. Myelography and CTM outline the intraspinal mass, which may extend to or through the dura, and even into the spinal cord.[9] Ocassionally, neither a prevertebral mass nor an anterior vertebral defect can be seen, and an isolated intraspinal cyst is present.[5]

DEVELOPMENTAL MASS LESIONS

Epidermoids and dermoids are considered to arise from intraspinal cell rests. The epidermoid derives from epithelium, whereas the dermoid derives from both epithelium and dermis. These cysts are three times more common in females than males, and occur most frequently in the lumbosacral region. The cysts are extramedullary in 60% of cases and intramedullary in 40%. A cutaneous dermal sinus is present in approximately 25% of dermoid cysts.[10] Except in the presence of a dermal sinus, the epidermoid and dermoid are not distinguishable radiographically. Those cysts involving the filum terminale are often small, producing only mild thickening of the filum. Cysts occurring above the filum tend to be bulkier, more discrete masses (Fig. 10).[22] Myelography shows

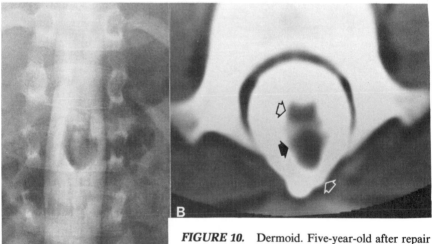

FIGURE 10.   Dermoid. Five-year-old after repair of lipomyelomeningocele. A, Myelogram shows a mass in the subarachnoid space adjacent to the conus at L1. B, CTM outlines an intradural extramedullary mass (open arrow) posterior to the conus (solid arrow). The mass shows a density similar to that of the conus, indicating that it is not a lipoma. At the same level is a small meningocele (white arrow).

the mass but cannot distinguish it from a lipoma. On CTM, a dermoid or epidermoid shows a density ranging from -30 to $+30$ Hounsfield units, whereas a lipoma shows a lower density of approximately -60 Hounsfield units.[29] CTM may also show the dermal sinus connecting to a dermoid.

Teratomas are rare congenital tumors containing derivatives of ectoderm, mesoderm, and endoderm. They may be intramedullary or extramedullary, and occur most frequently in the thoracic cord. Often large, a teratoma may extend over several vertebral lengths or even involve the entire spinal cord.[9] On myelography, the teratoma is indistinguishable from other developmental or neoplastic masses. On CTM, the teratoma may appear solid or cystic, and may show fatty components or calcification.[9]

Abnormal fatty deposits are found in the lipomyelomeningocele and in some cases of tethered cord. In addition, a lipoma may be present as a circumscribed intradural mass. Myelography shows an intradural mass lesion, but CTM shows the low density, and therefore fatty nature, of the mass.[9]

REFERENCES

1. Aubin ML, Vignaud J, Jardin C, Barr O: Computed tomography of 75 cases of syringomyelia. AJNR 2:199–204, 1981.
2. Barnes PD, Lester PD, Yamanashi WS, Prince Jr.: Magnetic resonance imaging in infants and children with spinal dysraphism. AJNR 7:465–472, 1986.
3. Barson AJ: The vertebral level of termination of the spinal cord during normal and abnormal development. J Anat 106:489–497, 1970.
4. Bentley JFR, Smith JR: Developmental posterior enteric remnants and spinal malformations: The split notochord syndrome. Arch Dis Child 135:76, 1960.
5. Blevins K, Buchino JJ, Fellows R: A child with chronic abdominal pain and leg weakness. J Pediatr 105:329–332, 1984.
6. Davis RL, Robertson DM: Textbook of Neuropathology. Baltimore, Williams & Wilkins, 1985, pp 192–193.
7. Fallon M, Gordon ARG, Lendrum AC: Mediastinal cysts of fore-gut origin associated with vertebral abnormalities. Br J Surg 41:520–533, 1954.
8. Fiske CE, Filly RA: Ultrasound evaluation of the normal and abnormal fetal neural axis. Radiol Clin North Am 20:285–296, 1982.
9. Fitz, CR: Congenital anomalies of the spine and spinal cord. In Computed Tomography of the Head, Neck and Spine. Chicago, Year Book Medical Publishers, 1985, pp 715–739.
10. Fitz, CR: Developmental Abnormalities of the Spine: The Clinical Neurosciences. New York, Churchill Livingstone, 1984, pp 827–847.
11. Fitz CR, Harwood-Nash DC: The tethered conus. Am J Roentgenol Radium Ther Nucl Med 125:515–523, 1975.
12. Garceau GJ: The filum terminale syndrome. J. Bone Joint Surg 35A:711–716, 1953.
13. Hawass ND, El-Badawi MG, Fatani JA, et al: Myelographic study of the spinal cord ascent during fetal development. AJNR 8:691–695, 1987.
14. Heinz ER, Rosenbaum AE, Scarfl TB, et al: Tethered spinal cord following meningomyelocele repair. Radiology 131:153–160, 1979.
15. Hilal SK, Marton D, Pollack E: Diastematomyelia in children. Radiology 112:609–621, 1974.
16. Jones PH, Love JG: Tight filum terminale. Arch Surg 73:556–566, 1956.
17. Kan S, Fox AJ, Vinuela F, Debrun G: Spinal cord size in syringomyelia: change with position on metrizamide myelography. Radiology 146:409–414, 1983.
18. Kan S, Fox AJ, Vinuella F: Delayed metrizamide CT enhancement of syringomyelia: postoperative observations. AJNR 6:613–616, 1985.
19. Kantrawitz LR, Pais MJ, Burnett K, Choi B, Pritz MB: Intraspinal neurenteric cyst containing gastric mucosa: CT and MR findings. Pediatr Radiol 16:324–327, 1986.
20. Kendall B: Iohexol in paediatric myelography, an open noncomparative trial. Neuroradiology 28:65–68, 1986.
21. Lee BCP, Zimmerman RD, Manning JJ, Deck MDF: MR imaging of syringomyelia and hydromyelia. AJNR 6:221–228, 1985.
22. Levine RS, Geremia GK, McNeill TW: CT Demonstration of cervical diastematomyelia. J Comput Assist Tomogr 9:592–594, 1985.

23. Lichenstein BW: "Spinal dysraphism" spina bifida and myelodysplasia. Arch Neurol Psychiatry 44:792–810, 1940.

24. Naidich TP, Fernbach SK, McLone DG, Shkolnik: Sonography of the caudal spin and back: congenital anomalies in children. AJNR 5:221–234, 1984.

25. Naidich TP, Harwood-Nash DC: Diastematomyelia: hemicord and meningeal sheaths; single and double arachnoid and dural tubes. AJNR 4:633–636, 1983.

26. Naidich TP, McLane DG, Mutluer S: A new understanding of dorsal dysraphism with lipoma (lipomyeloschisis): radiologic evaluation and surgical correction. AJR 140:1065–1078, 1983.

27. Neuhauser EBD, Harris GBC, Berrett A: Roentgenographic feature of neurogenic cysts. Am J Roentgenol Rad Ther Nucl Med 79:235–240, 1958.

28. Pettersson H, Fitz CR, Harwood-Nash DCF, Armstrong E, Chuang SH: Adverse reactions to myelography with metrizamide in infants, children, and adolescents: I. General and CNS effects. Acta Radiol Diagn 323–329, 1982. II. Local injury caused by lumbar puncture and injection of contrast medium. Acta Radiol Diagn 331–335, 1982.

29. Pettersson H, Harwood-Nash DCF: CT and Myelography of the Spine and Cord. New York, Springer-Verlag, 1982.

30. Pojunas K, Williams AL, Daniels DL, Haughton VM: Syringomyelia and hydromyelia: magnetic resonance evaluation. Radiology 153:679–683, 1984.

31. Roos RAC, Vielvoye GJ, Voormolen JHC, Peters ACB: Magnetic resonance imaging in occult spinal dysraphism. Pediatr Radiol 16:412–416, 1986.

32. Sarwar M, Virapongse C, Bhimani S: Primary tethered cord syndrome: a new hypothesis of its origin. AJNR 5:235–242, 1984.

33. Scheible W, James HE, Leopold GR, Hilton SvW: Occult spinal dysraphism in infants: screening with high-resolution real-time ultrasound. Radiology 146:743–746, 1983.

34. Scotti G, Musgrave MA, Harwood-Nash DC, et al: Diastematomyelia in children: metrizamide and CT metrizamide myelography. AJNR 1:403–410, 1980.

35. Sumner, TE, Crowe JE, Phelps, CR, Park RW: Occult anterior sacral meningocele. Am J Dis Child 134:385–386, 1980.

36. Thron A, Schroth G: Magnetic resonance imaging (MRI) of diastematomyelia. Neuroradiology 28:371–372, 1985.

37. Veeneklass GMH: Pathogenesis of intrathoracic gastrogenic cysts. Am J Dis Child 83:500–507, 1952.

38. Williams RA, Barth RA: In utero sonographic recognition of diastematomyelia. AJR 144:87–88, 1985.

JOHN BISESE, MD

EVALUATION OF SPINAL DYSRAPHISM BY MAGNETIC RESONANCE IMAGING

From the Department of Radiology, Georgia Baptist Hospital, Atlanta, Georgia

Reprint requests to:
John Bisese, MD
Department of Radiology
300 Boulevard, NE
Atlanta, GA 30312

The role of magnetic resonance imaging (MRI) in evaluating spinal dysraphism was reviewed in 50 patients, ages 3 months to 20 years. Diagnoses included the entire gamut of spinal dysraphisms. We have been impressed with the relative ease of satisfactory MRI evaluation of the entire craniospinal axis in patients with spinal dysraphisms.

METHOD

The usual imaging session was between 40 to 50 minutes. Patients in the pediatric age range were sedated with 30–50 mg/kg of chloralhydrate. In most cases, we were successful in obtaining satisfactory sagittal and axial examinations. The earlier cases were limited to the specific area in question, such as the lumbar sacral spine for evaluation of a myelomeningocele sac. As our experience grew, we attempted to include the entire neuroaxis and dropped the longer T2 spin echo sequences in favor of shorter, more complete T1-weighted examinations with short TRs. This change resulted in an increased amount of time.

GENERAL INFORMATION

In early embryogenesis, the spinal cord extends to the end of the spinal canal. Vertebral body growth exceeds that of the neural tissue and the cord appears to ascend. At birth, the conus lies at the L2–3 level and by 3 months at the L1–2 level. At maturity, the T2–L1 level is the usual location of the conus. The normal filum teminale extends through the tip of the thecal sac and attaches to the posterior aspect of the coccyx. The normal filum should measure less then 2 mm in diameter.

"Magnetic resonance imaging has proved to be a valuable adjunct in the study of children with spinal cord pathology. In the child with a history of a mye-lomeningocele, MRI has demonstrated tethered neural plaque lesion. Another intraspinal lesion that is quite frequent with children with myelomeningocele is the problem of hydromyelia. As is well known, MRI is the study of choice for the diagnosis of this lesion. At our institution it is believed that any child with a history of myelomeningocele should have a complete evaluation of his spinal cord, as over 90% of these children have associated lesions. Aside from the Arnold-Chiari malformation, other commonly seen lesions are the tethered neural plaque, hydromyelia, diastematomyelia, and intramedullary cyst." *(Mary M. Johnson, M.D., Pediatric Neurosurgery)*

Spinal Dysraphism

The common feature of a spinal dysraphism is an incomplete fusion of the posterior neural tube or the overlying bony structures. Spina bifida is a dysraphic state involving the bony vertebral column manifesting itself as a failure of the lamina and spinus processes to fuse in the midline. The dysraphisms involving the neural elements can be divided into two large groups. In his article in *Radiology* titled "Congenital pathology of the spine and spinal cord," Thomas Naidich classifies these groups by the presence or lack of skin closure over the defects. The first category (lack of skin closure) includes the myelomeningocele and myelocele. With closure of the skin, the defect is considered occult and includes the dorsal dermal sinus, simple meningoceles, anterior sacral menin-goceles and diastematomyelias.

Chiari's Classifications

Three classifications were established by Chiari in 1891 in his paper on hind brain dysgenesis. Chiari I is a simple displacement of the tonsils, possibly including the inferior vermis, into the upper cervical canal. Chiari II includes the tonsils and lower brain stem (medulla). The fourth ventricle is elongated and its inferior aspect extends through the foramen magnum. Chiari III is an extreme and rare anomaly. The entire cerebellar contents and lower brain stem are displaced through the foramen magnum and exit the cervical canal through a cervical spina bifida. The reason for including the Chiari anomalies with spinal dysraphism is the high association (100%) of the Chiari II malformation with myelomeningocele and hydrocephalus.

Chiari I (Figs. 1–3). An excellent article in AJR by Barkovich et al. (1986) used MR to study the position of the cerebellar tonsils and concluded that location of the lip of the tonsil up to 2 mm below the foramen magnum was within acceptable limits. Anything beyond this was felt to represent a Chiari I malformation. This can be a difficult clinical diagnosis and may often mimic a foramen magnum tumor or even multiple sclerosis. Although we have seen several cases of pediatric Chiari I, Barkovich et al. state that the diagnosis is often made in early or mid-adulthood. The associated findings of a Chiari I include the presence of a syringohydromyelia (50%), Klippel-Feil syndrome (37%), and cervicomedullary kinking (12%). Bands and adhesions have also been associated with this abnormality.

Chiari II (Figs. 4–9). Chiari II is associated with a myelomeningocele defect. There is a greater extrusion of both tonsil and brain stem into the cervical canal, which deforms and elongates the fourth ventricle. Associated findings of

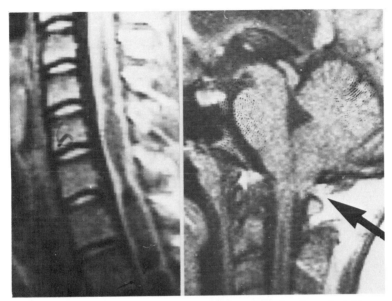

FIGURE 1. (*left*) A 15-year-old male with neck and head pain and right arm pain. The clinical question concerned a possible mass causing C7–T10 radiculopathy on the right.

FIGURE 2. (*right*) A 24-year-old female with known syringomyelia was referred to exclude glioma. Patient had left shoulder and neck pain, and right arm and shoulder pain extending into the hands.

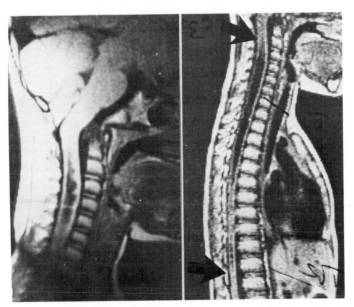

FIGURE 3. A 7-year-old with a 5-week history of right-sided leaning. No other problems were noted. The typical Chiari malformation and the extensive syrinx extending from the dens of C2–T12 are shown.

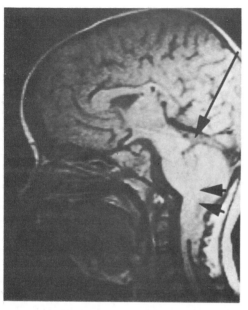

FIGURE 4. A 3-year-old patient with shunted hydrocephalus and myelomeningocele repair. Note the large amount of inferior displacement of the brain stem and tonsils as well as the very thinned fourth ventricle. Note the tectile plate beaking.

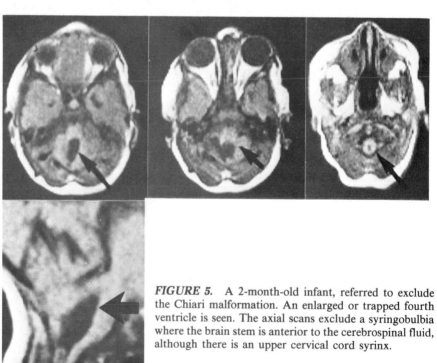

FIGURE 5. A 2-month-old infant, referred to exclude the Chiari malformation. An enlarged or trapped fourth ventricle is seen. The axial scans exclude a syringobulbia where the brain stem is anterior to the cerebrospinal fluid, although there is an upper cervical cord syrinx.

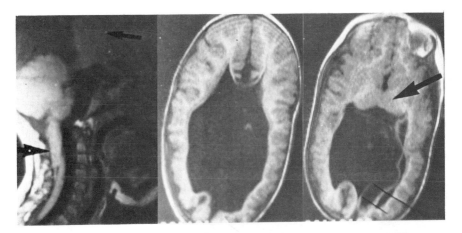

FIGURE 6. A 2½-year-old patient after shunt with a loss of grip and alertness. Note the associated agenesis of the corpus callosum with fused thalamic bodies and wide abnormal ventricles.

hydrocephalus, corpus collosal agenesis, and other forms of brain dysmorphia have been encountered with this abnormality.

Simple Meningoceles

These meningoceles (Fig. 10) contain no intrinsic neural tissue, and the enlarged thecal sac extends through a posterior spina bifida. This is one of the rarest forms of spinal dysraphism; the example illustrated is located in the thoracic region.

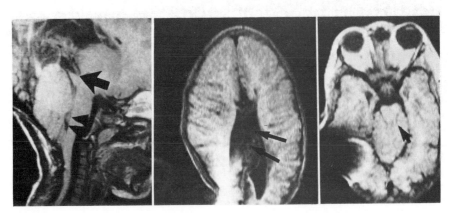

FIGURE 7. The Chiari malformation is seen in a 3-year-old female who had previous myelomeningocele repair. Note the inferior location and characteristic distortion of the fourth ventricle as well as the marked beaking of the tectile plate (arrow). The sagittal examination shows the absence of the corpus callosum. Axial images confirm the diagnosis. The ventricular appliance can be easily identified.

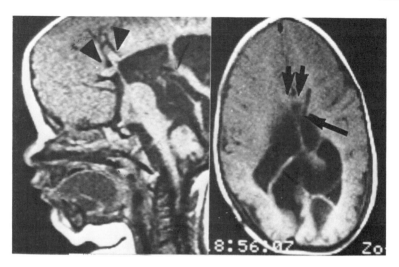

FIGURE 8. Chiari II with partial corpus collosal agenesis. Note preservation of the more anterior corpus callosum (arrows).

Syrinx (Figs. 11–15)

Hydrosyringomyelia represents fluid-filled spaces within the cord, either arising from a dilated central canal (hydromyelia) or outside the central canal (syringomyelia). There is a high association of hydrosyringomyelia with the Chiari malformation and myelomeningocele dysraphism. Magnetic resonance allows imaging the entire neural tube. Neurosurgical drainage tubes are not affected and are not a contraindication for imaging.

The pathogenic origin of syringomyelia in the Chiari malformation is generally felt to be related to pulsations of cerebrospinal fluid through the obex of the fourth ventricle. Gardner and Williams have both proposed a valve mechanism provided by the ectopically low tonsils that causes cerebrospinal fluid to flow through the obex, allowing the syrinx to be formed.

There are several classifications of syrinx, but the two commonest communicating (communication of the contral syrinx fluid cavity with the subarachnoid space) and noncommunicating. Syrinx may also be described as uncomplicated (communicating), traumatic, idiopathic, or syringomyelia associated with tumor. The cavity may vary in length from 1 to 17 vertebral segments. It is important to extend the area of MR coverage significantly above and below the syrinx cavity to include the entire cavity.

Septations have been seen in several cases, and may represent gliosis or fibrosis. The presence of residual communicating pathways may also account for the septations. Additionally, the gliosis or reaction of the neural tissue surrounding the syrinx shows increased signal on the more T2-weighted images, and at times differentiation from small tumors is difficult.

Diastematomyelia (Figs. 16 and 17)

Diastematomyelia is a striking abnormality, easily recognizable on MRI, particularly on coronal images. Diastematomyelia consists of a sagittal clefting

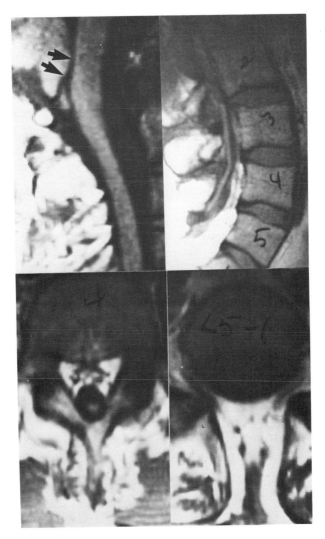

FIGURE 9. A 30-year-old male with spina bifida who has had repair of meningocele and now has exacerbation of low-back and left-leg pain.

of the cord, conus, or filum. The condition is seen predominantly in females. There is a 50–75% association with cutaneous stigmata. The most apparent characteristic is the fawn's tail or tuft of long hair over the lower lumbar sacral region, present in 60% of orthopedic abnormalities.

Plain films are an essential part of the diagnosis of diastematomyelia and usually show segmentation, hemivertebral bodies, or scoliosis. Examination of plain films is helpful in detecting a bony bar that may form the focus of cleft in the cord.

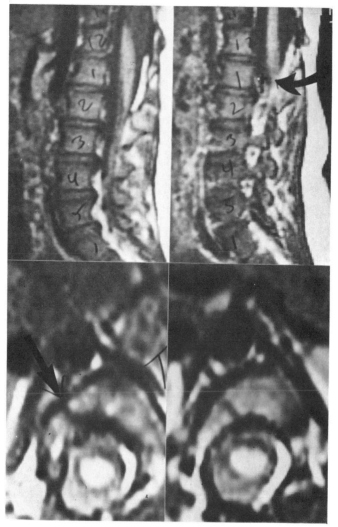

FIGURE 10. A 12-year-old female with a hairy patch over her midback, referred for evaluation of occult dysraphism.

Spina bifida occulta is usually present in 85–100% of these cases. The diastematomyelia is normally located in the lower thoracic region. Several diastematomyelia or more superiorly located diastematomyelia is rare and constitute 5% of this population.

The diastematomyelias can be divided into two groups. The first group shows duplication of the thecal sac; the second shows separate dural sacs for the hemicords. Tethering is associated in 75% of cases and a thick filum is identified in 90% of cases.

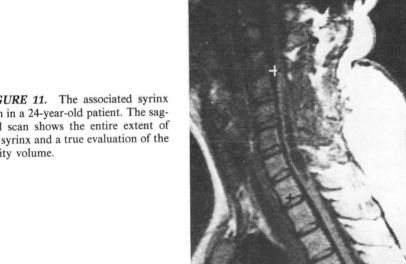

FIGURE 11. The associated syrinx seen in a 24-year-old patient. The sagittal scan shows the entire extent of the syrinx and a true evaluation of the cavity volume.

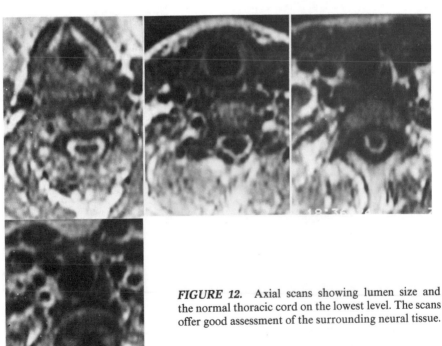

FIGURE 12. Axial scans showing lumen size and the normal thoracic cord on the lowest level. The scans offer good assessment of the surrounding neural tissue.

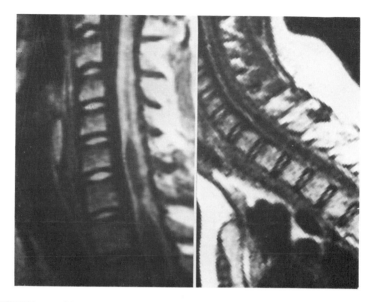

FIGURE 13. Note the ease with which the entire syrinx cavity can be shown.

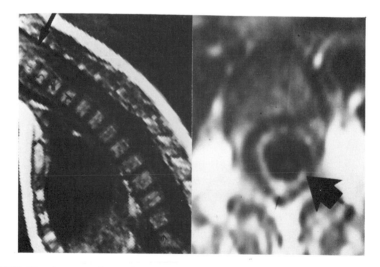

FIGURE 14. An extensive syrinx cavity associated with Chiari II and a myelomeningocele. Note the wrap-around artifact (arrow).

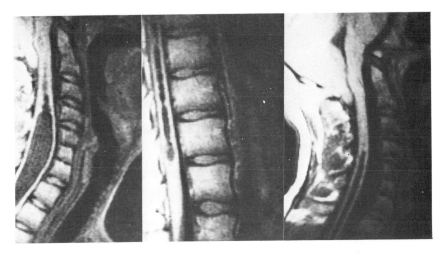

FIGURE 15.   Excellent follow-up of the treated syrinx can be obtained.

Tethered Spinal Cord (Figs. 18–21)

A tether is anything that fixes the spinal cord in an abnormally low location by either fibrous band, bone spurs or mass. The essential pathophysiologic characteristic is a stretching of the spinal cord that constricts, or puts at risk, the blood supply. Symptoms include paraparesis, paraplegia, sensory loss, and reduced bladder and bowel function.

A defect in the filum may indicate the filum terminale syndrome. This syndrome should be suspected when an abnormally thick filum is seen, and occurs in females in 57% of all cases. Symptoms are accelerated between the ages of 5–10 years and 10–15 years, and are thought to parallel growth spurts.

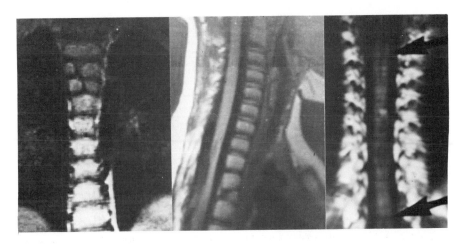

FIGURE 16.   This 3½-year-old male complaining of back pain and leg weakness had repair to meningocele.

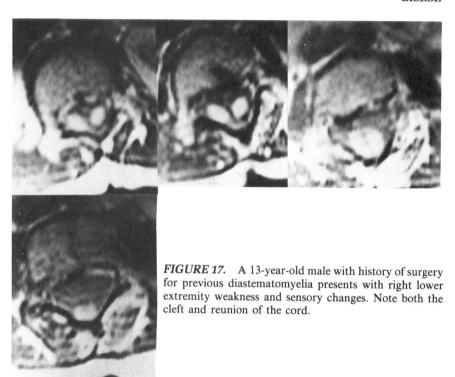

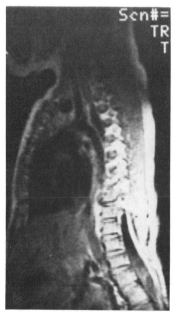

FIGURE 17. A 13-year-old male with history of surgery for previous diastematomyelia presents with right lower extremity weakness and sensory changes. Note both the cleft and reunion of the cord.

FIGURE 18. A 17-month-old female after myelomeningocele repair. There is a low cord insertion below the L2 level and a possible secondary area of tethering at the T10 level along the lowest present bony arch.

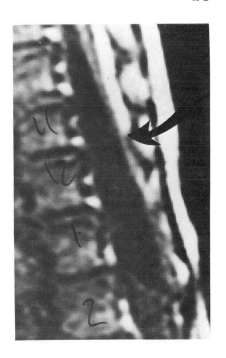

FIGURE 19. An 11-month-old male evaluated for hydromyelia. Patient is in a chronically flexed position. Note stretched attenuated cord that appears to be inserted at approximately the T11–T12 level under the T11 spinous process.

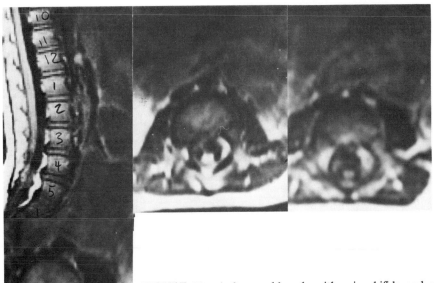

FIGURE 20. A 2-year-old male with spina bifida and a previous renal problem referred for evaluation of the lower spinal region to exclude cord tethering.

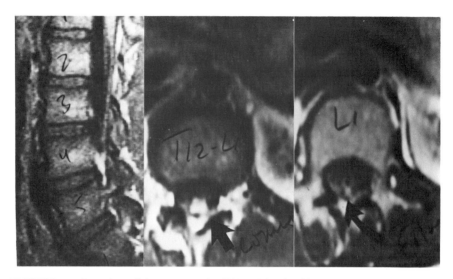

FIGURE 21.   Location of the conus at the T12–L1 level. This 11-year-old with scoliosis was examined to exclude an intradual abnormality of occult dysraphism.

In both cord and filum type tether, cutaneous stigmata are often the only clues to occult dysraphism. Features include midline skin dimple, hemangioma, or hypertrichosis; 17–25% of patients also have clinically apparent kyphoscoliosis.

Examination of plain films shows 100% of these patients to have spina bifida, usually a posterior bony defect at the L4–5 or L4–S1 level. The conus

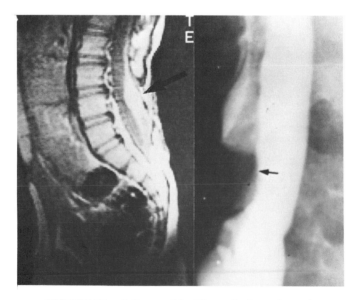

FIGURE 22.   A 3-year-old with repaired meningocele.

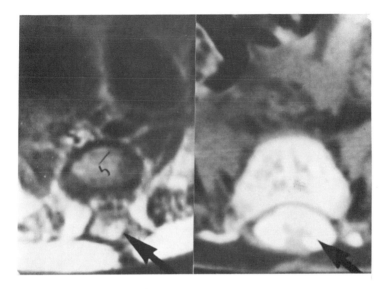

FIGURE 23. A 2½-year-old female with meningocele and cord repair. The thickened cord is closely applied to the posterior aspect of the canal.

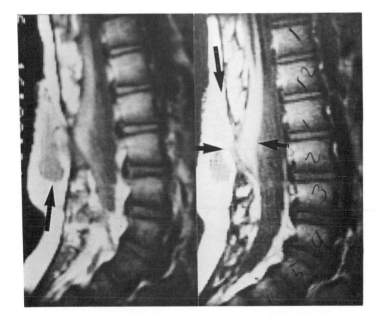

FIGURE 24. The meningocele sac is shown in the sagittal and axial orientation.

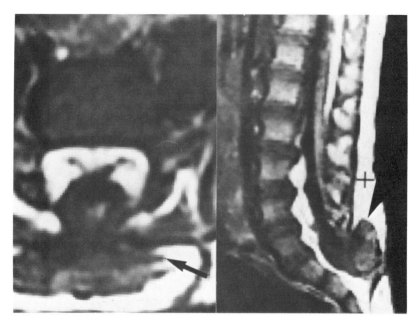

FIGURE 25. A 17-month-old with meningocele.

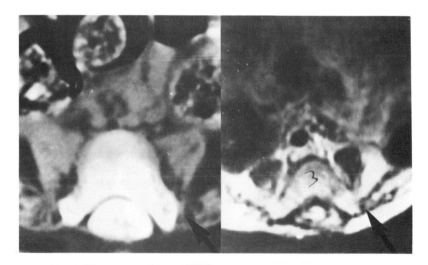

FIGURE 26. A 2½-year-old female with repaired myelomeningocele. Note the everted lamina.

is usually identified in an abnormally low position below L2. In 86% of patients with abnormally thick filum, there are approximately 30% that have a fibrolipoma involving or extending along the "thick filum." Another feature of the tethering syndrome is the tenting of the dura at the site of the abnormal attachment. This condition is probably related to where the filum has pierced the sac in an attempt to anchor itself.

Myelomeningocele

Myelocele.   Myelocele is a form of spina bifida in which the posterior aspect of the cord remains everted or splayed and flush against the midline posteriorly. The central portion of the defect represents a dysraphic cord that has failed to close posteriorly, and the peripheral portion consists of the meninges.

Meningocele.   A meningocele is a protrusion of cord or nerves covered by intact meninges through, but not covered by, the skin. In both cases (Figs. 22 to 25), 98% of the patients will have hydrocephalus and 80% will come to the attention of the orthopedic surgeon because of club foot, scoliosis, or congenital dislocation. A feature seen on CT, plain films, and MRI is the everted or abnormally separated pedical and laminar structures arrested in their attempt to close posteriorly.

Both hydromyelia and syringomyelia (Figs. 26 and 27) have a slight female predominance and increase in occurrence with Irish heritage. Plain films may show nearly normal to severely abnormal findings with hemivertebrae, segmentation, and numerous fusions. Because the basic defect is an absence of normal

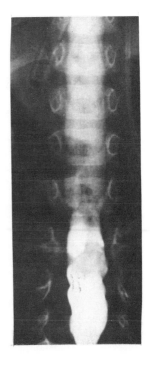

FIGURE 27. Associated findings with myelomeningocele. Hydromyelia and syringomyelia are seen in 10–77% of patients, diastematomyelia in 3–41%, and lipomas in 47%.

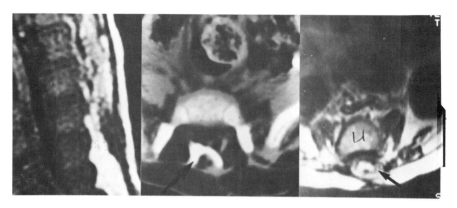

FIGURE 28. Two cases showing the fatty tumor on both the sagittal and axial images.

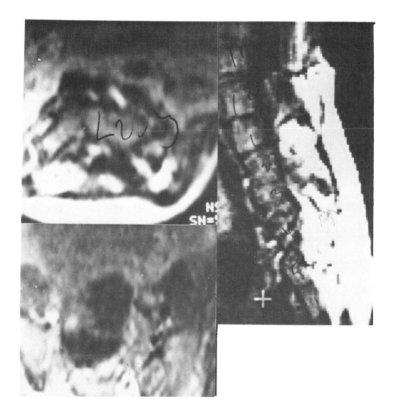

FIGURE 29. A 3-year-old female with problems walking. This is a preoperative evaluation before debulking of an intracanal lipoma.

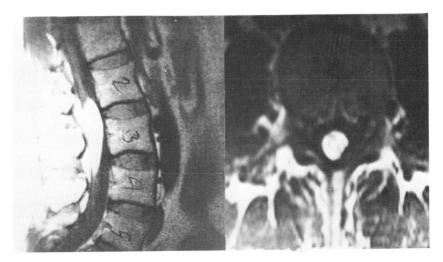

FIGURE 30. A 38-year-old with a 20-year history of left-sided problems and numbness and recent right-leg symptoms. Note the nerves passing through the high-signal-intensity fatty tumor.

posterior fusion, the elements remain everted with wide splaying of the lamina oriented in a posterolateral rather than posteromedial direction.

Lipomas (Figs. 28–30)

The lipomeningocele is the association of a myelomeningocele with a large fatty tumor. The cord shows a partial dorsal myeloschisis. The lipoma is intermittently adherent to the dorsal surface of the spinal cord along the cleavage. Cord and lipoma herniate through a wide spina bifida to form a dorsal subcutaneous mass. The tissue has the histologic characteristic of being fibrofatty.

The lipomyelomeningocele forms 60% of all occult spinal dysraphisms, and 50% of these have the cutaneous stigmata of the occult dysraphic syndromes.

A small subset of lipomas is the intradural lipoma, which forms less than 1% of all primary interspinal tumors.

CONCLUSION

Our initial experience has been rewarding with regard to the evaluation of spinal dysraphism. Magnetic resonance imaging offers an excellent alternative to CT and myelography, and the investment of time is considerably shorter. The advantages of MRI over ionizing forms of evaluation have been discussed. The multiplanar capacity has been shown to be of unique applicability in the spinal dysraphic syndromes.

It should be noted that successful images may not be obtained for all children in one session, and two or three sessions may be needed. This factor should not be a detraction, because myelography often requires hospitalization and anesthetic intervention.

In occult dysraphism, obvious dysraphism when indicated, and in the evaluation of scoliosis, MRI should be the method of choice after appropriate plain films have been obtained for proper evaluation of spinal dysraphism.

ALAN R. ALEXANDER, MD

MAGNETIC RESONANCE IMAGING OF THE SPINE AND SPINAL CORD TUMORS

From the Neuroradiology Division, Department of Radiology, St. Joseph Hospital, Lancaster, Pennsylvania

Reprint requests to:
Alan R. Alexander, MD
Department of Radiology
St. Joseph Hospital and
Health Care Center
250 College Avenue
Lancaster, PA 17604

Magnetic resonance imaging (MRI), in only a few years, has had a dramatic effect on the way many diseases are diagnosed. Its applications have grown exponentially with advancement of the technology, and its full impact is yet to be realized.

Until recently, evaluation of the spine and spinal cord for suspected tumors and other mass lesions has largely consisted of myelography and often exploratory surgery. Computed tomography (CT) represented a dramatic step toward an accurate and noninvasive method of evaluation of disease, but has a number of limitations, both technical and practical, and often requires intrathecal contrast. MRI now promises to largely replace both methods of evaluating tumors of the spinal cord and adjacent structures, and is currently considered by many authorities to be the modality of choice in evaluation of the spine and central nervous system.

GENERAL CONSIDERATIONS

The major advantages of MRI are numerous. The procedure is noninvasive and, except for occasional problems with the claustrophobic patient who may require sedation, is tolerated well by most patients. The entire length of the spinal cord and canal can be evaluated in multiple planes. There is no need for intrathecal contrast as MRI has superior soft tissue contrast. This allows for greater distinction between the spinal cord and subarachnoid space than is achievable by CT without intrathecal contrast.[6] There is no ionizing radiation and, at least currently, there are no known biological hazards.[2,13] There is also a lack of bone streak artifact that increases the ease of differentiating intramedullary from extramedullary lesions and provides superior definition of tumor cavities.

Current disadvantages include motion artifact, relatively poor capability for typing and grading of tumors, poor detection of calcification, and a potential for false-positive results.[3]

CLASSIFICATION OF TUMORS

For simplification purposes and also to aid in differential diagnosis, spinal cord tumors are classified into three main groups: intramedullary, extramedullary intradural, and extramedullary extradural.

Intramedullary Tumors

The superior resolution of the cord itself by MRI provides for easy differentiation of intramedullary from extramedullary masses. Intramedullary tumors represent approximately 15% of all spinal cord tumors.[11] The majority of these neoplasms are gliomas. The most common is ependymoma, which represents roughly 90%. The second most common glioma is the astrocytoma, which represents approximately 30%, followed by much lower incidences of the other gliomas, including oligodendroglioma and medulloblastoma. The remaining and relatively uncommon intramedullary tumors include hemangioblastoma, dermoid cyst, intramedullary lipoma, melanoma, and the rare nonneurogenic metastasis to the cord.[9] Several nonneoplastic processes include syringomyelia or hydromyelia, hematomas, and AVMs.

With the ability to do direct sagittal scans, the extent of tumor involvement is clearly depicted by MRI. Location of the lesion may be helpful in offering a logical differential diagnosis. For instance, ependymomas are more common at the conus level where they frequently present as a fusiform swelling of the filum terminale or as well-encapsulated nodules (Fig. 1). They may also occur in the

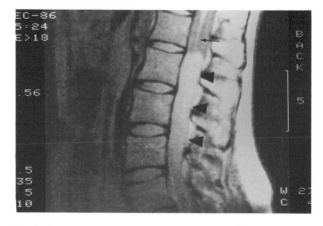

FIGURE 1. Typical appearance and location of an ependymoma, presenting as a large intradural mass (black arrowhead) just below the conus and closely associated with the filum terminale (small arrow).

cervical area. Astrocytomas most often occur in the cervical-thoracic region and are more common in children.[1]

The majority of tumors present as low to intermediate signal intensity lesions on T1-weighted scans and show differing degrees of increased signal intensity on more T2-weighted scans. Exceptions include hemorrhagic tumors and lipomas, which are typically bright on the T1-weighted scan.

Both astrocytomas and ependymomas can cavitate and form centrally cystic areas of degeneration (Fig. 2). The differentiation of cystic neoplasms from benign cysts may be difficult, but the combination of distinct margins and

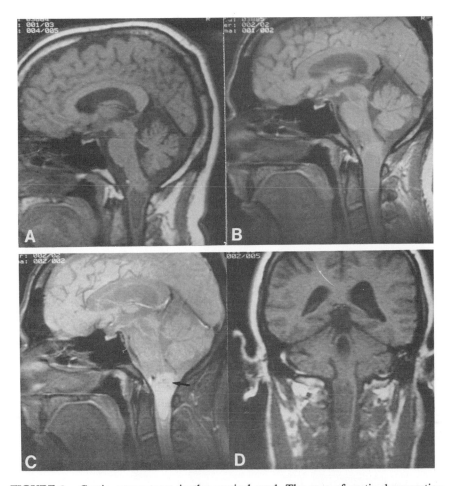

FIGURE 2. Cystic astrocytoma in the cervical cord. The area of cystic degeneration appears as a well-circumscribed area of low signal on the T1-weighted image (*A*), with increasingly brighter homogeneous signal on more T2-weighted scans (*B,C*). The irregular contour and signal behavior (small arrow) in the superior portion of the mass (*A–D*) is an area of solid tumor and differentiates this from a benign cyst.

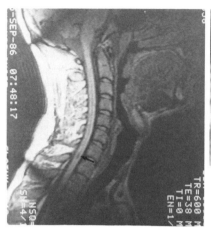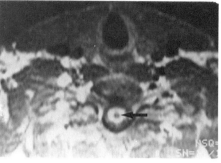

FIGURE 3. Post-traumatic syrinx of the cervical cord.

uniform signal intensity, equal to cerebrospinal fluid, is highly suggestive of spinal cord cysts (Fig. 3).[14] However, there is some overlap between cysts and cystic tumors. DiChiro et al.[3] report that the grading of primary cord tumors according to their signal characteristics has not been encouraging based on current technology and pulsing sequences. MRI of arteriovenous malformations (AVMs) has been discussed in the literature.[1,3] The serpiginous draining veins can sometimes be detected, although not consistently (Fig. 4). Differentiation of intramedullary versus extramedullary AVMs is more easily defined with MR than any other method, including arteriography and dynamic CT.[3]

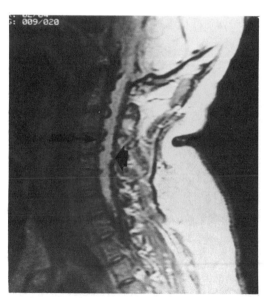

FIGURE 4. Serpiginous draining veins of a cervical dural arteriovenous malformation are clearly visible (arrow).

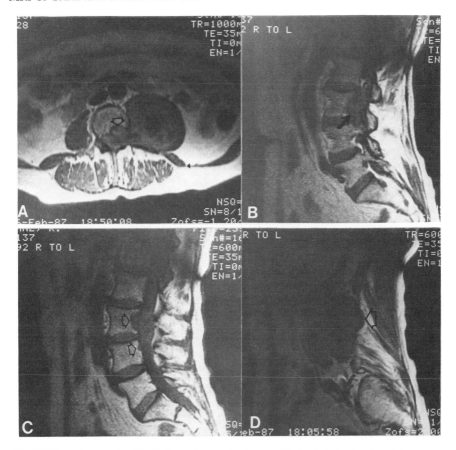

FIGURE 5. Large dumbbell thoracic meningioma with both intradural and large extradural components. *A–C*, Erosion of the adjacent pedicle and posterior aspect of the adjacent vertebral bodies (arrowheads). Tumor extension through the neural foramen is seen on both the axial and sagittal scan (black arrow, *B*). *D*, Large paraspinal component and its craniocaudal extent. A dumbbell neurofibroma would look much the same and could not be differentiated by its MR appearance.

Extramedullary Intradural Tumors

This is the most common group of spinal cord tumors, representing between 50% to 60% of spinal neoplasms. Most of these lesions are benign. By far, the commonest lesion is the meningioma, which accounts for between 25% to 45% of all spinal tumors.[8] Women are affected more often than men, showing a peak incidence in the fifth and sixth decades. The vast majority of spinal meningiomas are found in the thoracic region (Fig. 5), with cervical being the second most common location (Fig. 6, 7). These are primarily intradural extramedullary tumors, but can present as the classic "dumbbell tumor" with extension into the extradural compartment (Fig. 5). Their signal characteristics by MR are variable, although most are isointense to the adjacent spinal cord. The presence

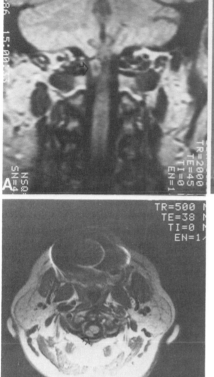

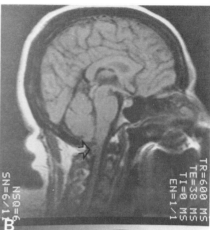

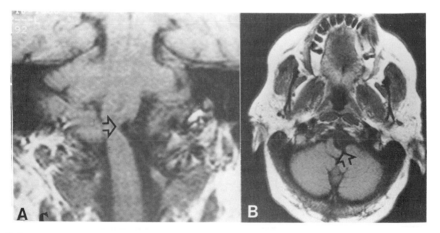

FIGURE 6. Coronal (*A*), sagittal (*B*), and axial scans (*C*) show a small meningioma at the level of the foramen magnum. Cord compression is clearly shown. Note how well the small tumor is shown without the problem of bony streak artifacts seen on CT.

FIGURE 7. Axial and coronal scans of a calcified foramen magnum meningioma showing marked signal dropoff.

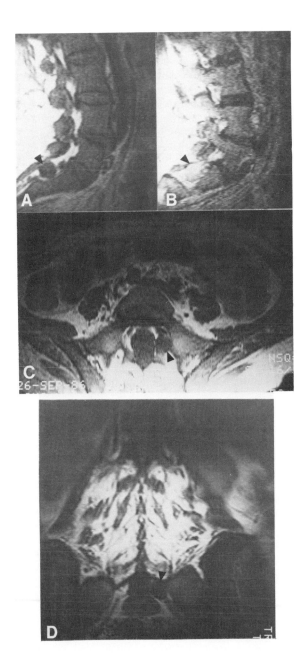

FIGURE 8. Neurilemmoma of the S2 root. *A,* T1-weighted sagittal scan shows a well-circumscribed mass eroding the back of the S1 vertebral body with isointense signal to adjacent nerves. *B,* T2 sagittal scan shows marked increase signal. *C* and *D,* Axial and coronal T1 images showing excellent anatomic delineation of the lesion and adjacent structures.

of calcification may lead to further dropoff of signal on both T1 and T2-weighted scans (Fig. 7).

The next most common group are the nerve sheath tumors, which include the schwannomas, neurilemmomas, and neurofibromas (Fig. 8). Neurilemmomas, unlike meningiomas, show no particular predilection as to sex or location. They can be variable in appearance and may be quite large. They may have both extradural and intradural components, presenting as the classic dumbbell tumor. These tumors have no specific signal characteristics by MR. Although the tumors are usually solitary, they are occasionally multiple. Whenever there is more than one, the possibility of generalized neurofibromatosis should be in the differential diagnosis.

Other, less common causes of an intradural extramedullary mass are intradural metastases, including drop metastases from primary tumors of the central nervous systems and also metastatic disease outside of the central nervous system, especially melanoma and bronchogenic carcinoma.[11] Occasional leptomeningeal involvement from lymphoma may present as intradural masses.

Extradural Tumors

Metastatic tumor is, by far, the most common cause of extradural tumors. This includes various blood-borne tumors, either directly to the epidural space or, more commonly, due to secondary invasion or spread to the epidural space from an involved vertebral body. The most frequent metastatic tumors to the spine include carcinoma of the breast, prostate, lung, and kidney, and other carcinomas. Other tumors include melanoma, sarcoma, Ewing's sarcoma, lymphoma, leukemia, and multiple myeloma, as well as neuroblastic tumors.[4,8] Benign extradural tumors include neurilemmoma (Fig. 8), meningioma, lipoma,

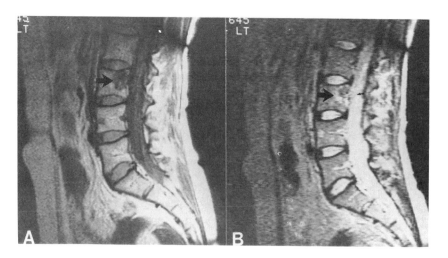

FIGURE 9. Metastatic breast carcinoma to the lumbar spine. *A,* T1-weighted scan shows normal bright signal of marrow in the vertebral bodies except for a large area of decreased signal in the L3 body (black arrow). A second smaller lesion is seen anteriorly in L4. *B,* T2 scan shows brightening of tumor deposits and signal dropoff of uninvolved marrow fat. Early epidural extension is also seen (small arrow).

dermoid, and epidermoid tumor. However, most tumors involving the extradural spaces are malignant.

Magnetic resonance is exquisitely sensitive in picking up changes within the vertebral bodies of marrow infiltration by tumor. This sensitivity is largely due to the very bright signal normally derived from marrow fat, which is typically bright on T1 images, with subsequent dropoff of signal on increasingly T2-weighted scans. When fat is replaced by tumor or other infiltrative processes, the normal fat signal is lost and, most typically, there will be an actual reversal of the normal signal characteristics in the involved segment of the vertebral body; it will be brightest on the T2-weighted scan (Fig. 9). The high signal contrast provided by the presence of fat makes MR sensitive to even small metastatic implants in the spinal column. An exception is the unusual circumstance where there is extensive diffuse marrow infiltration involving several adjacent vertebral bodies, but with preservation of normal architecture. On first glance, the scan may appear grossly normal, and the presence of metastatic

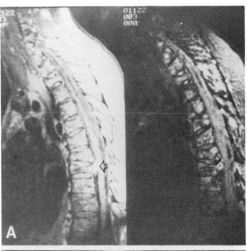
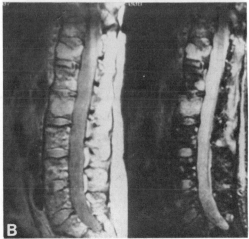

FIGURE 10. Sagittal proton density and T2-weighted image of the thoracic and lumbar spine in a patient with extensive breast carcinoma. Note how well the extent of disease is shown, including a pathologic compression fracture of a mid-thoracic vertebra with epidural tumor extension compressing the cord.

disease will be detected only if the reversal of normal signal characteristics is noted.

MRI has been reported to be as reliable as myelography, even when followed by CT, for the demonstration of subarachnoid space or spinal cord compression from epidural metastatic disease.[12] Smoker et al.[11] showed that MRI clearly identifies levels of blocks by tumor and, even in the absence of cord compression, effectively demonstrates subarachnoid space encroachment by epidural metastatic disease (Figs. 10 and 11).

Likewise, primary spinal and paraspinal masses are clearly delineated and their possible relationship to the intradural space, such as dumbbell tumors, (meningiomas, neurinomas, and neurofibromas), the largest component of which may well be extradural (Fig. 5).

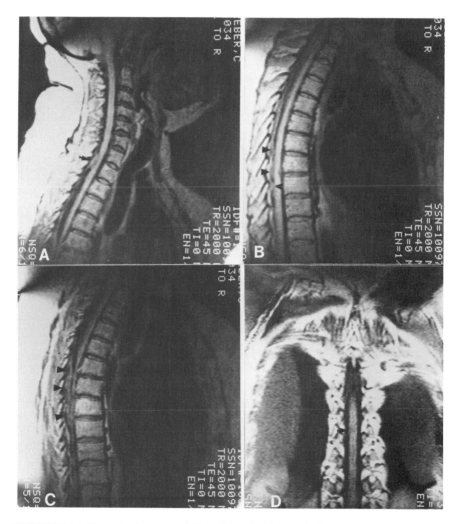

FIGURE 11. Extradural metastatic lymphoma in the cervical and thoracic spine. Note how clearly the tumor is shown to be in the extradural compartment.

CONCLUSION

Magnetic resonance imaging has many clear advantages over other available modalities in the evaluation of the spine and spinal cord for tumors and tumor-like conditions. These advantages include the ability to image large segments of the spine in multiple planes, with superior soft tissue contrast and sensitivity. This imaging can be accomplished without invasive procedures or intravenous contrast. MRI is highly sensitive in detecting and differentiating intramedullary, intradural extramedullary, and extradural masses of various etiologies. The current disadvantages include problems with motion artifacts, the inability to clearly type and grade tumors, and poor detection of calcifications. However, despite these disadvantages, MRI is considered to be the procedure of choice in the evaluation of various spinal and spinal cord pathologies and is largely supplanting computed tomography and myelography in their evaluation. Future developments in pulsing techniques and MR contrast agents will lead to further improvements and continued expansion of its clinical applications.

REFERENCES

1. Brant-Zawadski M, Norman D: Magentic Resonance Imaging of the Central Nervous System. New York Raven Press, 1987.
2. Budinger TF: NMR in vivo studies: Known thresholds for health effects. JCAT 5:800–811, 1981.
3. DiChiro, Giovanini et al: Tumors and arteriovenous malformations of the spinal cord: Assessment using MR. RAD 156:689–697.
4. Fischer MS: Lumbar spine metastasis in cervical carcinoma. A characteristic pattern. RAD 34:631–634, 1980.
5. Goy AMC, et al: Intramedullary spinal cord tumors: MR imaging with emphasis on associated cysts. RAD 161:381–386, 1986.
6. Han JS, et al: Radiol Clin North Am 22:805, 1984.
7. Holtas SL, Kido DK, Simon JH: MR imaging of spinal lymphoma. JCAT 10:111–115, 1986.
8. Newton TH, Potts DG: Modern Neuroradiology, Vol 1. Computed Tomography of the Spine and Spinal Cord. Clavadel Press, 1983.
9. Post MJD, Quencer RM, Green BA, et al: Intramedullary spinal cord metastases, mainly of non-neurogenic origin. AJNR 8:339–346, 1987.
10. Rubin JM, Aisen AM, DiPietro MA: Ambiguities in MR imaging of tumoral cysts in the spinal cord. JCAT 10:395–398, 1986.
11. Shapiro, Robert: Mylography. Chicago, Yearbook Medical Publishers, Inc. 1975.
12. Smoker WRK, et al: The role of MR imaging in evaluating metastatic spinal disease. AJNR 8:901–908, 1987.
13. Thomas JG, Morris PG: The effects of NMR exposure on living organisms. I. A microbial essay. Br J Radiol 54:615–621, 1981.
14. William AL, et al: Differentiation of intramedullary neoplasms and cyst by MR. AJNR 8:527–532, 1987.

WILLIAM W. WOODRUFF, JR, MD
Major, USAF, MC

EVALUATION OF DISC DISEASE BY MAGNETIC RESONANCE IMAGING

From the Department of Radiology,
Wilford Hall USAF Medical Center,
Lackland Air Force Base, Texas

Reprint requests to:
Major William W. Woodruff, Jr. MD
Department of Radiology
Wilford Hall USAF Medical Center
Lackland AFB, TX 78236-5300

The opinions or assertions contained here are the private views of the author and are not to be construed as official nor as reflecting the views of the United States Air Force.

Since the first image of the vertebral column was obtained late in the last century, the radiologist has played an increasing role in the evaluation of patients with disc disease. To image the disc and its perimeter, epidural venography, myelography and discography were developed. Significant complication rates were reported due to technical aspects of the procedures as well as reactions to and side effects from contrast material.

By 1973, computed tomography (CT) was introduced to the United States and revolutionized the evaluation of disc disease. This technique permits transaxial evaluation of contents of the spinal canal based on differences in the attenuation coefficient of the contents within a given volume of tissue. However, unenhanced CT may be of limited use in the evaluation of disc disease in the thoracic, and to a lesser extent, the lower cervical canal due to beam hardening artifacts and lack of significant differences in the attenuation coefficients of the canal contents at these levels. However, with the use of water-soluble intrathecal contrast, CT is often used in conjunction with myelography to permit more complete evaluation of the cord, spinal canal, and its perimeter, including the intervertebral discs.

Magnetic resonance imaging (MRI) is the most recent addition to the radiographic armamentarium and represents an evolutionary advance in the evaluation of disc disease. Using slight differences in the proton density, and T1 and T2 relaxation times of various tissues, MRI allows multiplanar visualization of discs, cerebrospinal fluid, cord, and the perimeter of the spinal canal without the use of intravenous contrast.

ANATOMY

On T1-weighted images (T1-WI; short TR–short TE), the typical vertebral body consists of a central region of relatively high-signal intensity representing fat within the marrow cavity (Fig. 1). The signal intensity of the marrow cavity is approximately equal to or slightly greater than that of adjacent skeletal muscle. Cortical bone is seen as a perimeter of decreased signal intensity due to the lack of mobile hydrogen protons. The posterior elements, including the pedicles, articular facets, lamina, and spinous process, also contain a marrow space of high-signal intensity surrounded by cortical bone of low-signal intensity that may be seen on parasagittal and axial T1-WI.

The appearance of the disc on T1-WI has been described.[4] The central portion of the disc representing the nucleus pulposus and the annulus fibrosus are indistinguishable from one another. Collectively, the signal intensity of this central region is slightly hyperintense to the more peripherally located collagen (Sharpey's) fibers. On parasagittal T1-WI, a band of signal void composed of the opposing vertebral body endplate and disc margin is identified. Frequently the signal void along the inferior disc margin is wider than that from the superior disc margin. This is secondary to a chemical shift artifact occurring in the frequency encoded direction and is not related to an actual increase in the thickness of the cortical bone.

The canal contents are well visualized on T1-WI. Cerebrospinal fluid has a long T1 relaxation time and a low-signal intensity. Parasagittal and axial images obtained throughout the level of the cord demonstrate good delineation between the CSF and the higher-signal intensity cord. On the parasagittal images, the transition from conus to cauda equina is often indistinct and may require augmentation with axial images at the appropriate level. Epidural fat has high-signal intensity and may be found throughout the ventral aspect of the spinal canal, increasing in amount in a caudal direction. Epidural fat is consistently present in the intervertebral foramen and provides excellent contrast as it surrounds the exiting spinal nerves of lower-signal intensity. Signal void from epidural veins may be identified on T1-weighted parasagittal images within the ventrally located epidural fat, particularly in the lumbar region.

As a result of the increased acquisition time for the T2-weighted images (T2-WI; long TR–long TE), there is often a dramatic decrease in the quality or resolution of an image. In addition to patient motion (particularly degrading in the thoracic spine from respiratory and diaphragm motion), there is a dramatic decrease in the signal-to-noise ratio. This results in a set of images that may appear to be aesthetically unappealing, yet contain valuable diagnostic information (Fig. 1).

On T2-WI, the signal intensity of the marrow cavity decreases relative to that on T1-WI. The signal intensity of the cortical bone remains lower than the fat-ladened cancellous bone with a detectable difference between their signal intensities in the body and posterior elements.

The normal disc has a central region of high-signal intensity on T2-WI, representing the nucleus pulposus and annulus fibrosus. The collagen fibers in the periphery of the disc are of slightly lower-signal intensity.[4] Often present in the central portion of the disc is a band-like region of decreased signal intensity. Aguila et al.[1] have ascribed this to an intranuclear cleft frequently present in normal discs in patients over 30 years of age.

The boundary of the subarachnoid space is well visualized on both parasagittal and axial images. The high-signal intensity of the cerebrospinal fluid on T2-WI, however, obscures the fine definition of the cord and cauda. The signal

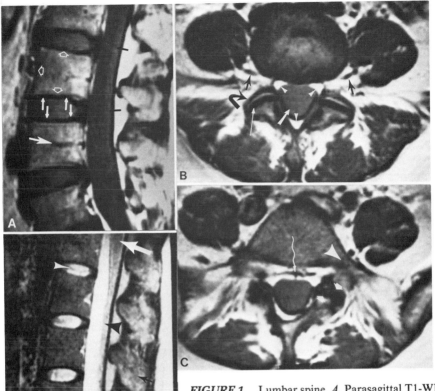

FIGURE 1. Lumbar spine. *A*, Parasagittal T1-WI showing normal alignment and signal intensity of the vertebral bodies. The linear region of decreased signal intensity within the central portion of the vertebral bodies (large arrow) indicates the path of the basivertebral veins. Note the decreased signal perimeter of the vertebral body representing the dense cortical bone (open arrows). The L3–4 disc shows the normal decreased signal intensity of the collagen fibers and opposing vertebral body endplates both cephalad and caudad to the disc (small arrows). Incidentally, a bulging disc is present at the L4–5 level. The cauda equina (black arrows) is of slightly greater signal intensity than the surrounding cerebrospinal fluid. *B*, Axial T1-WI at the L5–S1 disc space shows the thecal sac (arrow) surrounded by epidural fat (arrowheads). The L5 ganglion is identified (black arrows) bilaterally, anterior lateral to the intervertebral foramina. The superior articular facet of S1 (curved black arrow) is located anterior lateral to the inferior articular facet of L5 (long white arrow). *C*, Axial T1-WI just caudal to the disc space shows the pedicles of S1 (arrowhead) and the most inferior extent of the L5–S1 articular facet joints (short arrow) bilaterally. The epidural venous plexus (undulating arrow) is identified juxtaposed between the S1 body and the thecal sac. *D*, Parasagittal T2-WI in a different patient showing normal alignment and signal intensity of the vertebral bodies. The spinous processes (black arrows) are clearly depicted. The discs at the upper three lumbar levels are normal. The intranuclear cleft (white arrowhead) is identified. Note the decreased signal arising from the L4–5 and L5–S1 level (small white arrows) secondary to desiccation. The conus (large white arrow) is well visualized with the cauda equina (black arrowhead) slightly obscured by the cerebrospinal fluid of higher-signal intensity.

513

intensity of the epidural fat decreases on T2-WI, rendering the intervertebral foramen and its contents slightly less distinct than on the T1-WI.

CERVICAL SPINE

Unique to the cervical spine are the Luschka joints (Fig. 2). These joints contain the uncinate processes that extend superiorly from the posterior portion of the vertebral body below to articulate with depressions in the posterior inferior portion of the vertebral body above. Luschka joints are a frequent site of involvement in cervical spondylosis. The pedicles are directed in a lateral-posterior orientation and the articular facets are more horizontal in orientation. The craniocervical junction including the foramen magnum, cerebellar tonsils, and cervical cord, as well as the atlanto-axial articulations, are well visualized on axial and parasagittal images.

On T1-WI, high signal intensity material within the ventral posterior vertebral body cortex and the more dorsal CSF. This material also surrounds the exiting spinal nerve as it courses through the neural foramen. Although this shortening of T1 relaxation time has been ascribed to adipose tissue, autopsy studies[2] have shown a paucity of fat. Rather, a rich venous network has been identified in these anatomic regions. The flow-related enhancement has been implicated as the cause of this high signal intensity.

THORACIC SPINE

There is progressive increase in height and width of the vertebral bodies from a cranial to caudad direction (Fig. 3). Also, the pedicles arise from the more dorsal aspect of the vertebral body and extend posteriorly. The dimensions of the canal increase in caudal progression.

LUMBAR SPINE

In response to chronic weight-bearing in the biped, the vertebral bodies, posterior elements, and discs increase to their maximum size in the lumbar spine, with the L4–5 disc space usually being the widest. The articular facets have become nearly completely vertical in orientation. The area of the spinal canal increases to its maximum.

PATHOLOGY

Degenerative Disc Disease

Degeneration of the disc may occur in a continuum ranging from desiccation of the disc to marked annular bulging or herniation of the nucleus pulposus. Our imaging is done over a relatively static period which may occur anywhere within this spectrum. Alternatively, disc disease may not represent a predictable progression and may be precipitated by a significant mechanical force.

For this report, degenerative disc disease will refer to disc desiccation, annular bulges, prolapsed disc (subligamentous herniated nucleus pulposus), and herniated nucleus pulposus with or without a free fragment.

Desiccation of the disc occurs as the disc undergoes early degenerative changes; T2-WI are most sensitive at showing the decreased signal intensity resulting from desiccation of the disc. This early degenerative change may also be a central subtle region of decreased signal intensity on T1-WI.

As the nucleus pulposus degenerates and the annulus fibrosus weakens, the axial loading pressure compresses the disc (Fig. 4). As a secondary feature, the annulus begins to bulge. The bulge most frequently occurs symmetric throughout

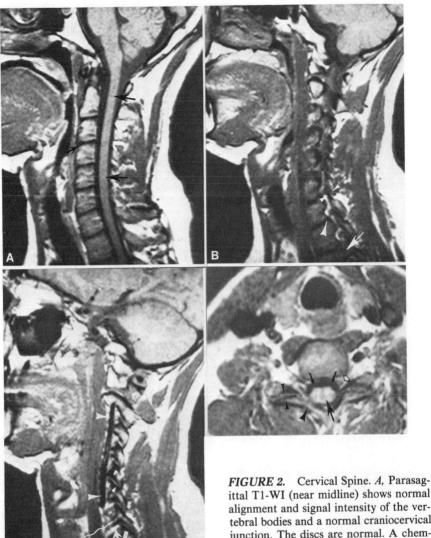

FIGURE 2. Cervical Spine. *A,* Parasagittal T1-WI (near midline) shows normal
alignment and signal intensity of the vertebral bodies and a normal craniocervical
junction. The discs are normal. A chemical shift artifact accounts for the conspicuous decreased signal arising from the
disc and superior vertebral body margins
(small arrow). The cord (large arrows) is well visualized as it is surrounded by relative
decreased signal from the cerebrospinal fluid. *B,* Parasagittal T1-WI 5 mm lateral to Fig.
2A shows the osseous elements of the spinal canal including the uncinate process (large
arrowhead), pedicles (arrow), and the most medial extent of the articular facets (small
arrowheads). *C,* Parasagittal T1-WI 5 mm lateral to Fig. 2B shows the vertebral artery
(large arrowheads) within the foramen transversarium. Pedicles (undulating arrow),
articular facets (small arrowheads), and material of high signal intensity within the
intervertebral foramen (curved arrows) are well seen. *D,* Axial T1-WI at the level of the
C5–6 intervertebral foramen shows the cord (large arrow) surrounded by lower intensity
cerebrospinal fluid (small arrows). The relatively higher-signal intensity material within
the foramen provides contrast to evaluate the exiting C6 roots of lower-signal intensity
(open arrow). Articular facets (small arrowheads) and lamina (large arrowhead) are
seen clearly.

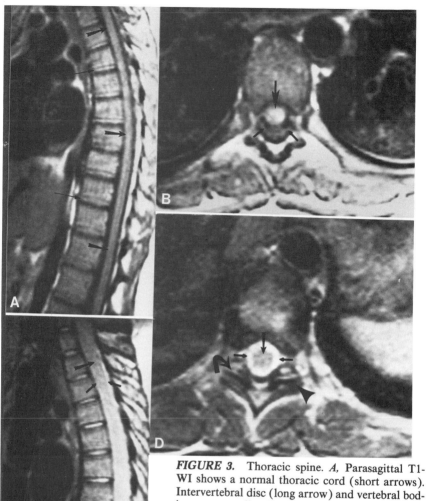

FIGURE 3. Thoracic spine. *A,* Parasagittal T1-WI shows a normal thoracic cord (short arrows). Intervertebral disc (long arrow) and vertebral bodies are normally aligned and of normal signal intensity. The subarachnoid space is identified ventral and dorsal to the cord. *B,* Axial T1-WI of the lower thoracic spine shows a normal bony perimeter of the spinal canal. The cord (long arrow) is of slightly greater signal intensity than the surrounding cerebrospinal fluid within the subarachnoid space (short arrows). *C,* Parasagittal T2-WI shows the cerebrospinal fluid and cord to be of nearly equal signal intensity where the spinal cord is nearest to the surface coil. As the thoracic kyphosis moves the canal contents deep to the surface coil, the cord and fluid interface becomes more conspicuous with the cerebrospinal fluid (short arrows) maintaining a higher-signal intensity than the cord (long arrows). The signal intensity of a midthoracic disc is decreased (white arrow) relative to other discs, representing desiccation of the disc. Otherwise the discs and vertebral bodies are normal. *D,* Axial T2-WI shows good delineation between the more central cord (long arrow) and surrounding cerebrospinal fluid (short arrow). The bony perimeter of the spinal canal is normal. The superior articular facets (curved arrow) are easily distinguishable from inferior articular facets (arrowhead) at this level.

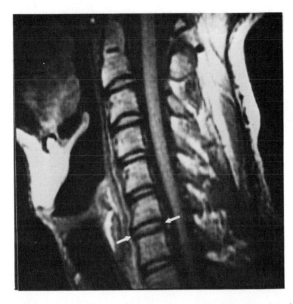

FIGURE 4. Bulging cervical disc. Parasagittal T1-WI showing symmetric extension of the disc beyond the anterior and posterior margins of the vertebral bodies at the C6–C7 level (arrows).

the disc space in all directions. The annulus, however remains intact. Commensurate narrowing of the disc space will occur reflecting the decreased vertical dimension of the degenerative disc. With MRI, the bulge is easily identified as the disc extends beyond the signal void cortical bone of the vertebral body above and below the disc. The degree of extension of the bulging disc into the spinal canal may be detected on parasagittal and axial T1-WI. However, due to the relatively greater difference in the T2 relaxation times, between the desiccated disc and the cerebrospinal fluid, T2-WI may be necessary to define this interface. The degree of compromise of the neural foramen may be adequately evaluated with axial T1-WI as the epidural fat surrounding the exiting nerve becomes effaced.

A prolapsed disc occurs when a small amount of nucleus pulposus herniates through a focal defect in the annulus fibrosus. The herniated material, however, is separated from the dural sac by an intact posterior longitudinal ligament. Prolapsed discs usually occur posteriorly. Parasagittal and axial T1-WI adequately show the abnormality. A defect on the subarachnoid space is usually absent. The ventral epidural fat may remain intact. The epidural fat and exiting nerve root within the neural foramen remain normal. It is unlikely that T2-WI will be useful in absence of any defect on the thecal sac.

A herniated disc occurs when material from the nucleus pulposus extends through a defect in the annulus fibrosus (Fig. 5). This typically occurs posteriorly or posterolaterally, yet less frequently may also occur in a lateral direction (Fig. 6). A free fragment occurs when the herniated nucleus pulposus loses its contiguity with the native disc. The herniated disc material may be shown on parasagittal and axial T1-WI particularly if the epidural fat of high-signal in-

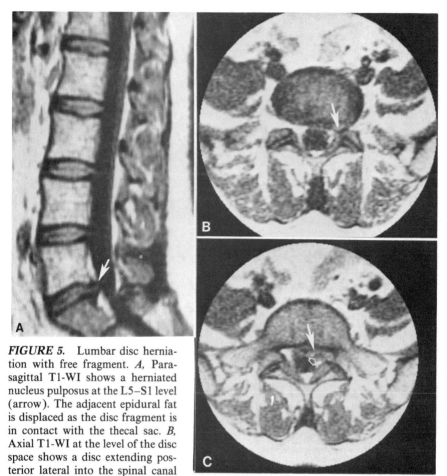

FIGURE 5. Lumbar disc herniation with free fragment. *A,* Parasagittal T1-WI shows a herniated
nucleus pulposus at the L5–S1 level
(arrow). The adjacent epidural fat
is displaced as the disc fragment is
in contact with the thecal sac. *B,*
Axial T1-WI at the level of the disc
space shows a disc extending posterior lateral into the spinal canal
and proximal neural foramen (arrow). The epidural fat is effaced. *C,* Five millimeters
caudal to the disc space a free fragment is present in the spinal canal (arrow) displacing
the left SI root (open arrow) as it effaces the surrounding epidural fat.

tensity or veins are effaced. The actual defect on the thecal sac is more conspicuous on T2-WI.

Spondylosis

Spondylosis is a degenerative process involving the intervertebral disc, the
vertebral bodies, and the various ligamentous structures that line the spinal
canal. Spondylosis occurs as a broad clinical and radiographic spectrum from
involvement of single disc level without canal stenosis to multilevel disease with
significant central canal stenosis and possible underlying cord atrophy.

The disc often undergoes degenerative changes with varying degrees of disc
bulge and disc space narrowing. The narrowing of the disc space allows the
normally taut ligamentum flavum to become redundant and protrude into the
spinal canal, decreasing the area of the canal dorsally. Disc changes are frequently

accompanied by bony changes. Osteophytes may project into the canal from either the inferior or superior margins of the dorsal aspect of the vertebral body. The articular facets may undergo bony overgrowth with resultant lateral recess or neural foramen stenosis.

The discs, osteophytes, and ligaments are well demonstrated on T1-WI (Figs. 7, 8). Cord atrophy and distortion may be identified on T1-WI. The T2-WI may be useful to detect the amount of narrowing of the subarachnoid space and thus the degree of canal stenosis.

The vacuum disc may occur in a disc that has undergone severe degenerative changes. This accumulation of nitrogen gas within the disc results in an area of signal void usually contained by the annulus fibrosus. Grenier et al.[3] have found the T1-WI parasagittal images most useful in demonstrating this abnormality.

Frequently the radiographic abnormalities are unrelated to the patient's clinical appearance. Teresi et al.[6] reported the MRI findings in 100 asymptomatic patients with degenerative disc disease of cervical spondylosis. All patients were under evaluation for head and neck tumors. The frequency of cervical spondylosis including disc herniation or bulge, osteophyte formation, cord impingement, and cord herniation increased with age. Concave defects in the ventral subarachnoid space secondary to disc disease or osteophyte formation occurred in 16% and 26% of patients less than 64 years of age or greater than 64 years of age, respectively. A detectable concave defect in the cord was identified in 7% of their patient population.

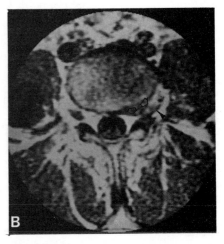

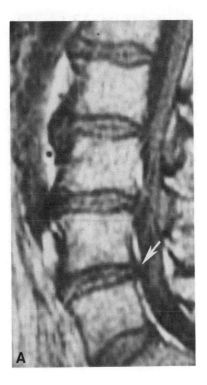

FIGURE 6. Lateral lumbar disc. *A*, Parasagittal T1-WI near the level of the L4–L5 neural foramen shows a subtle mass (arrow) isointense to the disc extending posterior and lateral into the spinal canal. *B*, Axial T1-WI obtained at the L4–L5 disc space shows an isointense mass (open arrows) representing a true lateral disc filling the neural foramen and displacing the left L4 ganglion (arrowheads).

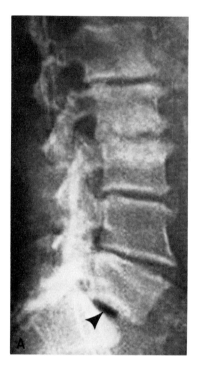

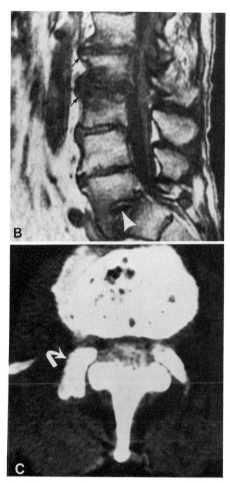

FIGURE 7. Spondylosis—vacuum disc. *A,* Lateral digital scout view shows marked degenerative changes of the lumbar space with disc space narrowing throughout, and a vacuum disc at L5–S1 (arrowhead). Marked reactive bony changes are identified at L1–2 and L2–3. *B,* Parasagittal T1-WI showing similar finding with vacuum disc (arrowhead) as a region of signal void. Regions of decreased signal intensity are identified at the level of and extending anterior to the L1–2 and L2–3 disc spaces representing hypertrophic bony changes (arrows). Bulging discs are seen at all levels. *C,* CT after myelography of L2–3 shows advanced degenerative changes with sclerosis of the endplate and a bulging disc with mild canal stenosis. Moderate overgrowth of the superior articular facets of L3 is noted (arrow). *D,* Axial T1-WI through the L2–3 disc space shows central canal stenosis, overgrowth of superior articular facets of L3 (arrows), and decreased signal intensity along disc space representing the sclerosis and osteophyte formation (undulating arrows). *E,* Axial CT after myelogram at L5–S1 shows a vacuum disc (long arrow) and marked bony degenerative changes at the endplates and articular facets of S1 (short arrow). No evidence of central canal stenosis is identified. *F,* Axial T1-WI through the L5–S1 disc space with signal void representing vacuum disc (curved arrow). The normal appearance of the S1 articular facets is disrupted due to bony degenerative changes (straight arrows).

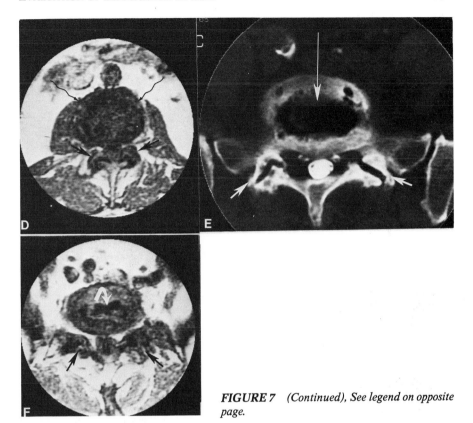

FIGURE 7 *(Continued), See legend on opposite page.*

Infection

Discitis may occur in response to various causes including surgical manipulation and trauma, and idiopathic causes. The inoculation may occur in the disc or adjacent vertebral body. In either case, the disc offers little resistance to the spread of the organisms, thus permitting contiguous involvement of the next vertebral body. As the organism multiplies and leukocytes begin to accumulate, the disc and vertebral body undergo destruction at a rate contingent on the virulence of the organism and the magnitude of the leukocyte response. An inflammatory mass consisting of portions of destroyed bone and disc as well as products of the leukocyte response begins to form.

On the T1-WI, the interface between the cortical bone and the adjacent collagenous disc fibers become less distinct (Fig. 9). Over time, the disc and disc space become completely obliterated. As cells infiltrate the cancellous bone and fluid accumulates, the normally high-signal intense marrow is displaced, leading to a decrease in the signal intensity within the vertebral body. The inflammatory mass has a generally low-signal intensity on T1-WI and may be seen as it displaces the epidural fat and veins within the spinal canal and neural foramina.

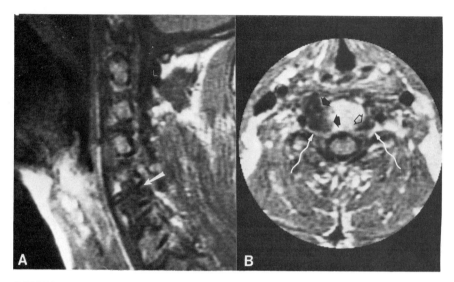

FIGURE 8. Cervical spondylosis. *A,* Parasagittal T1-WI through the right uncinate process shows generalized decreased signal intensity in region of Luschka joint at C5–6 (arrow) secondary to hypertrophic bony changes. *B,* Axial T1-WI at the C5–6 level confirms the bony changes on the right with prominent signal void from the cortical bone and loss of the Luschka joint space (black arrows). The material of high-signal intensity within the neural foramen (undulating arrows) is displaced by the bony reaction. The perimeter of the left intervertebral foramen is affected to a lesser degree (open arrow).

On T2-WI the edema and inflammatory reaction now have relatively high signal intensity. The extension of this material into the vertebral body is easily seen. Loss of the intranuclear cleft has been reported in patients with discitis.[1] Extension of the inflammatory mass into the prevertebral and paravertebral regions is clearly depicted due to the difference in signal intensity of the mass and adjacent skeletal muscle.

Tumor

Neoplastic processes rarely involve the disc. However, involvement of the vertebral column is frequently seen in patients with metastatic disease. The tumor may infiltrate the pedicles or vertebral bodies, creating soft tissue masses that compress exiting nerve roots or the spinal cord. In the right clinical setting, the effect on the central or peripheral nervous system may mimic the findings of disc disease.

The infiltration of neoplastic tissue into the cancellous bone will displace the normally high signal intense marrow on T1-WI (Figs. 10, 11). As the tumor extends through the bone, the signal void of the cortex will become interrupted. Tumor extension into the spinal canal may be easily assessed on T1- and T2-WI, obviating the need for myelography.[5] Frequently, the parasagittal MR images will demonstrate an early osseous metastatic focus, not apparent on myelography. This finding would be clinically useful when the occult osseous metastasis would not be included in the palliative radiation field.

PROTOCOL

Our current protocol for imaging disc disease includes parasagittal and axial T1 and T2-WI. The axial images are obtained parallel to the disc space. The decision to obtain axial images depends on the patient's suspected clinical level as well as abnormalities identified on parasagittal images. Parasagittal images alone are insufficient to evaluate for disc disease.

Currently spin echo sequences are most commonly used to obtain MR images. The T1-WI are obtained with a TR of 500 msec and TE less than 40 msec. The T2-WI are done with a TR of 1.5 to 2 sec and a TE of 40 to 100 msec. All images are 5 mm thick. Surface coils must be used in all spine work due to the need for greater resolution.

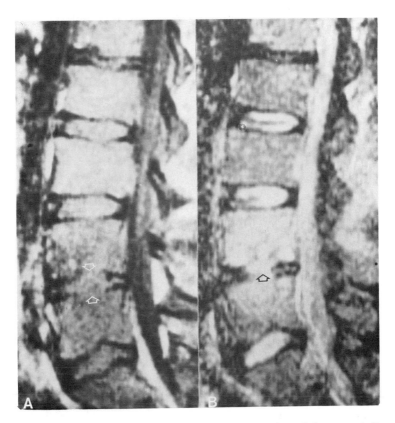

FIGURE 9. Discitis. *A*, Parasagittal T1-WI shows disruption of the normal disc space at the L4–5 level. Signal void from the opposing endplates is absent (arrows) indicating destruction. Disc space narrowing is present at the L4–L5 level. There is a subtle decrease in the signal intensity of the marrow cavity due to the infiltrative inflammatory process. *B*, Parasagittal T2-WI shows more clearly the degree of infiltration of the inflammatory process within the vertebral body as material of high-signal intensity replaces the normal marrow contents at both the L4 and L5 levels. Note the loss of the intranucleate cleft at the L4–L5 level (arrow). On the images, there is no evidence of extension into the spinal canal.

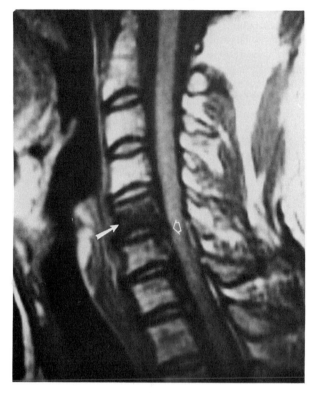

FIGURE 10. Metastatic breast tumor. Parasagittal T1-WI image shows replacement of the normal marrow of high-signal intensity by infiltrative tumor at the C5 body (arrow). A small amount of tumor extends into the canal and indents the ventral surface of the cord (open arrow).

New imaging protocols are being developed that use more narrow flip angles of the hydrogen protons. One advantage to this fast field echo technique is a decrease in the amount of time for data acquisition. Additionally, the narrow flip angle images allow a greater delineation between the cerebrospinal fluid of high-signal intensity and the spinal cord of lower-signal intensity (Figs. 12, 13).

CONCLUSION

Magnetic resonance is on the forefront of medical imaging. The application of MRI represents a quantum leap in our ability to evaluate patients with disc disease. Improved tissue sensitivity permits direct visualization of the disc and the contents of the spinal canal, obviating in many cases the need for more invasive contrast procedures.

ACKNOWLEDGMENTS

The author wishes to thank Naomi Jordan for her superb assistance with manuscript preparations. Also, Figures 1, 2, 3, 12, and 13 are courtesy of Philips Medical Imaging Systems, Inc.

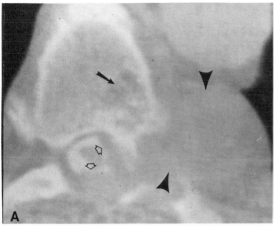
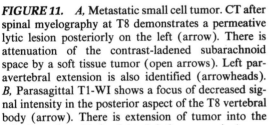
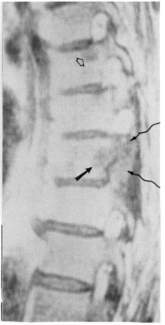

FIGURE 11. *A,* Metastatic small cell tumor. CT after spinal myelography at T8 demonstrates a permeative lytic lesion posteriorly on the left (arrow). There is attenuation of the contrast-ladened subarachnoid space by a soft tissue tumor (open arrows). Left paravertebral extension is also identified (arrowheads). *B,* Parasagittal T1-WI shows a focus of decreased signal intensity in the posterior aspect of the T8 vertebral body (arrow). There is extension of tumor into the spinal canal at this level (undulating arrows). A second occult lesion is noted at the T6 level (open arrow).

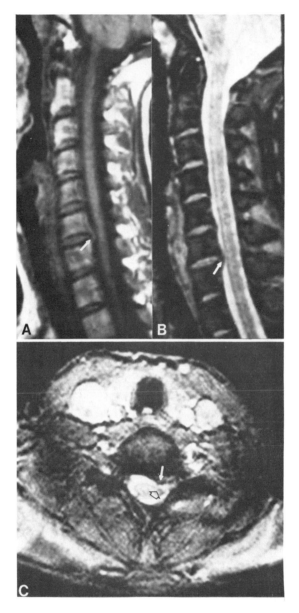

FIGURE 12. Cervical disc (fast field echo). *A,* The T1-WI (TR 450/TE 20) parasagittal show a herniated nucleus pulposus at C6–7 (arrow). The disc minimally deforms the ventral surface of the cord. *B,* Parasagittal fast-field echo image (TR 243/TE 14/Tip angle 7) more clearly identifies the ventral defect on the subarachnoid space (arrow). The cord, although not apparently deformed, is displaced posteriorly with narrowing of the dorsal subarachnoid space. There is excellent delineation of the cord within the subarachnoid space. *C,* Axial fast-field echo image at C6–7 shows a soft tissue mass (arrow) within the spinal canal causing asymmetric attenuation of the ventral subarachnoid space. Also, the cord deformity (open arrow) becomes apparent on axial images.

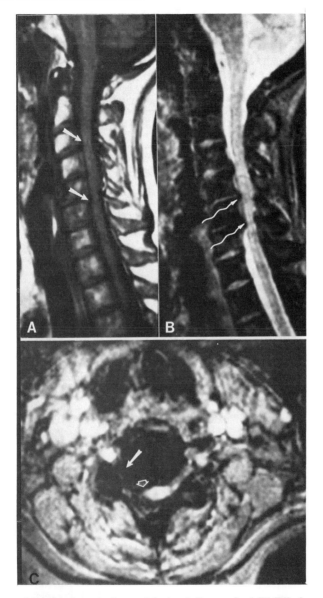

FIGURE 13. Multilevel cervical spondylosis. *A,* Parasagittal T1-WI shows loss of the normal lordotic curve of the cervical spine. The cord is deformed and posteriorly displaced from C4–C5 (arrows). Loss of the subarachnoid space ventral and dorsal to the cord indicates central canal stenosis. *B,* Parasagittal fast-field echo images confirm the degenerative disc disease with loss or decreased signal intensity of the disc at C3–4, C4–5, and C5–6. Ventral extradural defects are present at each of these levels. The cord is markedly deformed at C4–5 and C5–6 (arrows) with central canal stenosis. *C,* Axial fast-field echo image at C5–6 shows hypertrophy of the uncinate process and articular facets bilaterally, right greater than left (arrow). Also, a large osteophyte (open arrow) extends into the spinal canal on the right, with commensurate narrowing of the spinal canal. Marked central canal stenosis is present with the maximum dimension of the spinal canal less than 7 mm.

REFERENCES

1. Aguila LA, Piraino DW, Modic MT, et al: The intranuclear cleft of the intervertebral disk: Magnetic resonance imaging. Radiology 155:155–158, 1985.
2. Flannigan BD, Lufkin RB, McGlade C, et al: MR imaging of the cervical spine: Neurovascular anatomy. AJNR 8:27–32, 1987.
3. Grenier N, Grossman RI, Schiebler ML, et al: Degenerative lumbar disk disease. Pitfalls and usefulness of MR imaging in detection of vacuum phenomena. Radiology 164:861–865, 1987.
4. Pech P, Haughton VM: Lumbar intervertebral disk: correlative MR and anatomic study. Radiology 156:699–701, 1985.
5. Smoker WRK, Godersky JC, Knutzon RK, et al: The role of MR imaging in evaluating metastatic spinal disease. AJNR 8:901–909, 1987.
6. Teresi LM, Lufkin RB, Reicher MA, et al: Asymptomatic degenerative disk disease and spondylosis of the cervical spine: MR imaging. Radiology 164:83–88, 1987.

INDEX

Entries in **boldface type** indicate complete chapters.